NEUROSURGERY

NEUROSURGERY
An Introductory Text

Peter McLaren Black, M.D., Ph.D.
Franc D. Ingraham Professor of Neurosurgery
Harvard Medical School
Neurosurgeon-in-Chief
Brigham and Women's Hospital
Children's Hospital, Boston

Eugene Rossitch, Jr., M.D.
Assistant Professor of Neurosurgery
Harvard Medical School
Attending Neurosurgeon
Brigham and Women's Hospital
Children's Hospital, Boston

New York   Oxford
OXFORD UNIVERSITY PRESS
1995

Oxford University Press

Oxford   New York
Athens   Auckland   Bangkok   Bombay
Calcutta   Capetown   Dar es Salaam   Delhi
Florence   Hong Kong   Istanbul   Karachi
Kualu Lumpur   Madras   Madrid   Melbourne
Mexico City   Nairobi   Paris   Singapore
Taipei   Tokyo   Toronto

and associated companies in
Berlin   Ibadan

Copyright © 1995 by Oxford University Press, Inc.

Published by Oxford University Press, Inc.,
200 Madison Avenue, New York, New York 10016

Oxford is a registered trademark of Oxford University Press

Library of Congress Cataloging-in-Publication Data

Black, Peter McL.
Neurosurgery : an introductory text / Peter McL. Black, Eugene
Rossitch, Jr.
p.   cm.
Includes bibliographical references and index.
ISBN 0-19-504448-7 (cloth).—ISBN 0-19-504449-5 (paper)
1. Nervous system—Surgery.   I. Rossitch, Eugene.   II. Title.
[DNLM: 1. Neurosurgery—methods.   WL 368 B627h 1995]
RD593.B56   1995
617.4'8—dc20
DNLM/DLC   94-31469
for Library of Congress

9 8 7 6 5 4 3 2 1

Printed in the United States of America
on acid-free paper

PREFACE

Neurosurgical problems are not rare. Strokes, neck or back pain, head injury, seizures, spinal trauma, and headache are examples of relatively common complaints that may have neurosurgical implications.

We wrote this book to present the neurosurgical management of these and other conditions to non-neurosurgeons—to medical students, neurology or surgery residents, internists, and primary care physicians who want a concise introduction to this important field. We have emphasized practical diagnosis and management of neurosurgical disorders, beginning with chapters on the physical examination, imaging, symptom complexes, and differential diagnosis of common problems. We next discuss the management of emergencies, of non-emergent operative cases, and of neurosurgical medications, including a brief description of surgical procedures. After this we turn to neurosurgical conditions themselves—trauma of spine and brain, tumors, vascular disorders, disorders of cerebrospinal fluid, spine disorders, pediatric neurosurgery, epilepsy, and functional neurosurgery. In the last section we summarize cerebral neurological conditions that may mimic neurosurgical diseases.

We believe this text is a brief but complete introduction to neurosurgery. We hope readers will come away with the same affection for this exciting surgical discipline that we have.

Boston   P. McL. B.
May 1994   E.R., Jr.

ACKNOWLEDGMENTS

We would like to thank a number of neurosurgical trainees who have helped in the preparation of this book including Matthew Moore, Patrick Juneau, Steven Gelbard, P. Langham Gleason, Philip Starr, and Sumeer Sathi. We also are indebted to many other students, residents, and staff members, who have provided input on specific chapters.

We are also indebted to our colleagues at the Brigham and Women's and Children's Hospital—students, residents, and staff members—who have read specific chapters or otherwise given advice and encouragement. These include especially our neurosurgical colleagues, John Shillito, Michael Scott, Eben Alexander III, Philip Stieg, Joseph Madsen, and Lily Goumnerova.

Finally, we would like to thank Jeffrey House of Oxford University Press for his patient encouragement and advice.

CONTENTS

I

Neurosurgical Diagnosis

This section presents four aspects of diagnosis in neurosurgery: the clinical examination, including the history and physical examination and their abnormalities; imaging procedures, including "plain" X-rays, computed tomographic (CT) scans, and magnetic resonance imaging (MRI); various physiologic tests, including the electroencephalogram (EEG), positron emission tomography (PET) scanning, and single photon emission tomography (SPECT) scanning; and the differential diagnosis of common symptoms, including headache, weakness, sensory loss, neck and arm pain, leg pain, drowsiness, stroke, and dizziness. It is intended to provide a brief overview of the diagnostic arm of contemporary neurosurgery.

1

Clinical Diagnosis in Neurosurgery

Diagnosis in neurosurgery usually involves three steps: the organization of historical features and physical findings into syndrome complexes (syndrome identification), the identification of the anatomical region involved (anatomic diagnosis), and the clarification of the disease represented in a particular patient (etiological and pathological diagnosis). There is an old saying in neurology: "the history tells what the disease is and the examination tells where it is." Accurate diagnosis is a crucial initial step in neurosurgery.

In this chapter we will discuss the history and physical findings in neurosurgery, then present several important symptom clusters.

History

A careful history is as crucial in neurosurgery as in any other branch of medicine. In medicine the patient is sometimes approached as a series of specific problems, with relevant past history and physical findings considered under each problem. Although it is very helpful to summarize the patient's difficulties in this way at the end of the history and examination, it may be cumbersome to do this from the beginning of the history; any system that fully evaluates the patient is satisfactory. The history should include the patient's own idea of why he or she is seeking help, his or her account of symptoms including their nature, duration, exacerbating and relieving factors, related symptoms or events, a brief summary of past illnesses with

3

special attention to any previous surgical procedures and attendant problems, a list of drug or other allergies and precisely how they manifest themselves, an exact list of the medications the patient is taking and their frequency, and a review of systems that should be complete in the asking but succinct in the recording, noting those systems where problems occur.

The Physical Examination in Adults

The physical examination begins with a general examination, including blood pressure, pulse, temperature, respiration, height, and weight. These should be measured and not guessed at. Some statement should be made about the patient in general: whether withdrawn, agitated, obese, and so on. Details of how to do the chest, heart, abdominal, and extremity examination are available in general physical examination texts and will not be discussed here. Neck stiffness, head circumference, and carotid bruits are important aspects of the general examination sometimes overlooked.

Often a great deal of information about how the patient views the illness and the physician comes through in the examination, and this facet of the encounter should be explicitly recorded, since it can provide clues about cortical function as well as important information about the patient's expectations and understanding.

The Neurological Examination in Adults

The neurological examination should be thorough but not exhausting for either patient or physician. The chief goals are to characterize and localize abnormalities. The components of the neurological examination include cranial nerve, motor, reflex, sensory, cerebellar, mental status, and speech testing.

Cranial nerve examination begins with the first or olfactory nerve. This is best tested by holding cloves or coffee under each nostril. Ammonia is astringent and does not activate the olfactory bulb; it is sometimes useful if malingering is suspected because failure to perceive ammonia is not a defect of olfaction alone.

Evaluation of the optic nerve (II) involves funduscopic, visual field, and visual acuity examinations with an ophthalmoscope in a

on. If defects are found, more detailed te
scribed in specialty texts.

xamination in Infants and Young Childr

ological examination is based on the stage
. Several reflexes found in a newborn sho
hree months: these include the sucking refle
hen a lip is stroked; the grasp reflex, an in
he fingers placed in the palm; and the Moro
on of the arms when the child is suddenly l
held supine. The plantar reflex may rem
o age 2 or 3 years. Limb tone is an import
examination, providing clues about possi
ities.

t landmarks in development are as follows
llowed with the eyes at 12 weeks, sitting w
at 24 weeks, and crawling and standing shou
eeks. Walking and speaking have quite variat
re present in 90 percent of children by 14 and
y.

ested in an infant by using a moving object
y observing the response to a loud noise. T
can be plotted accurately on a percentile char
onth child should have a head circumference
th child 41–46 cm, a 12-month child 44–49 cn
d 46–52 cm.

he Neurological Examination

anosmia) may result from local disease in the
nic nasal infection, polyps, or tumor. The most
wever, is an old injury of the olfactory tract. A
oma or another tumor compressing the olfactory
se anosmia.

darkened room. The optic disc itself is examined for pallor or blurring of the disc margins, the retina for hemorrhage or exudates, and the retinal vessels for venous pulsations, narrowing or atherosclerosis. A long-distance (20 feet) eye chart should be used for acuity; a near-vision card is a less sensitive test. The visual fields are named temporal (to the side) and nasal (toward the nose) as the patient sees them. To test the fields, a 5-mm white object such as a pinhead is gradually brought into the upper or lower nasal or temporal field of one eye at a time.

The oculomotor, trochlear, and abducens nerves (III, IV, VI) are tested together by examining convergence (looking at one's nose), vertical and lateral eye movements, coordination of eye movements, lid droop, and pupillary size and reactivity. These functions reflect not only the cranial nerves but also the brainstem regions that contain their nuclei and the tracts that connect and influence them.

The trigeminal (V) nerve has both sensory and motor functions and three divisions. Pin and light touch should be tested over the forehead (V1), cheek (V2), and chin (V3); the corneal reflex tests V1 and the nostril tickle V2. Deviation of the jaw to either side tests the motor division of the trigeminal nerve: the motor root of the right trigeminal nerve supplies the right masseter muscle, making deviation of jaw to the left difficult.

Functions of the facial nerve (VII) include facial motion, taste in the anterior two-thirds of the tongue, salivation, tearing, sensation of the inner ear and tonsils, and stapedius muscle innervation. The nerve is tested by asking the patient to smile, frown, and pucker, and by testing perception of salt and sugar on the anterior tongue. An enlarged palpebral fissure can be a subtle sign of facial muscle weakness.

Testing of the auditory nerve (VIII) begins by making certain that the ear canals are free of wax, then whispering in one ear while scratching on a card held beside the other to block its hearing. If a whisper cannot be heard 12 inches from the ear, there is hearing loss. The next step is to assess whether the loss is conductive or neural; for this, a 512 cps tuning fork is held against the mastoid process and then held up to the ear after the patient has stopped hearing it. If the patient can hear the fork again, this is a normal or "positive" Rinné (air conduction is better than bone conduction). If there is conductive hearing loss, the fork will still not be heard. A second test to distinguish conductive from sensorineural loss is the Weber test. For this, a vibrating tuning fork is placed at the center of the forehead: with conductive loss from middle ear disease, the sound will be heard in the deaf ear better; with sensorineural loss it will be louder in the good ear.

The glossopharyngeal nerve (IX) is tested by noting symmetry of uvula movement and sensation in the pharynx (gag reflex). The accessory nerve (XI) is tested by asking the patient to turn his or her chin against the examiner's hand; a defective left nerve will make turning to the right weak.

The hypoglossal (XII) nerve is tested by evaluating the tongue for midline position and fasciculations. With a weak left XII nerve the tongue will deviate to the left on extension.

Motor testing begins with examination of muscle groups for atrophy, involuntary movements, or fasciculations (small rippling under the skin). Each muscle group listed in Table 1.1 should be tested by the corresponding maneuvers. Strength is graded from 0 to 5 as follows: 0- no contraction, 1- trace contraction, 2- movement that does not overcome gravity, 3- active movement against gravity, 4- active movement against resistance, 5- full strength. Tone is also estimated to be normal, increased, or decreased.

Table 1.1. Muscle Function and Innervation

Muscle	Movement	Major Root	Nerve
deltoid	arm elevation	C5	axillary
biceps	forearm flexion	C6	musculocutaneous
triceps	forearm extension	C7	radial
extensor carpi ulnaris	wrist extension	C7	posterior interosseous
opponens pollicus	thumb opposition	C8	median
finger flexors (pip joint)	grasp	C8	median
dorsal interossei	spreading fingers	T1	ulnar
iliopsoas	hip flexion	L2	femoral
quadriceps	leg extension	L3	femoral
tibialis anterior	foot dorsiflexion	L5	deep peroneal
extensor hallicus	great toe dorsiflexion	L5	deep peroneal
gluteus maximus	hip extension	L5	inferior gluteal
hamstrings	leg flexion	S1	sciatic
gastrocnemius	foot plantar flexion	S1	tibial nerve

Optic (II)

The optic nerve may demonstrate abnormalities on funduscopic examination, in visual acuity, or in visual field. On funduscopic examination, the normal optic disc is pink and well-demarcated with visible venous pulsations. The most important fundoscopic abnormality to recognize is papilledema—swelling of the optic nerve head that results from blockage to axoplasmic flow. The edges of the entire disc become indistinct. Central veins become engorged and nonpulsatile, and hemorrhages may develop as well as exudates in the retina. Papilledema is caused by increased intracranial pressure or arterial hypertension. There is usually no visual acuity loss except an enlarged blind spot. This feature differentiates it from optic neuritis, in which visual loss from a central scotoma may be severe. It often takes expert help to make the differential diagnosis between true papilledema and such conditions as optic drusen and pseudopapilledema. If there is doubt, consult a neuro-ophthalmologist. Untreated papilledema can progress to optic atrophy and blindness.

In *optic atrophy* the disc is pale and sharp; this always represents disease of the optic nerve or chiasm. Multiple sclerosis with optic neuritis, primary optic nerve tumors such as meningiomas or gliomas, tumors directly compressing the optic nerve or chiasm such as pituitary tumors or suprasellar meningiomas, central retinal artery occlusion, old glaucoma or papilledema, methyl alcohol intoxication, and some drugs can cause optic atrophy. In children, cerebromacular degeneration is also a possible cause.

Numerous problems may lead to *loss of visual acuity,* including corneal, lenticular, and retinal disorders and intracranial disease. Acuity loss from intracranial disease is usually accompanied by a visual field defect. Loss of acuity in one eye means disease of the optic nerve or orbit. A bitemporal loss suggests chiasmal compression, usually from a pituitary tumor.

Visual field testing is done either by moving spherical objects such as the head of a pin into view or by diminishing the brightness of lights kept stationary. Visual field evaluation can provide valuable information about diseases of the optic nerve and tracts. In reading fields, the middle of the field as displayed is perpendicular to the macula; the temporal field (70°) is wider than nasal (50°), and fields are presented as though you were looking at them; field deficits are described as nasal or temoral and upper or lower.

Three field patterns imply retinal disease: an arcuate defect from central retinal artery ischemia, an inferior hemianopia in one eye suggesting a vascular lesion, and an enlarged blind spot caused by an enlarged optic disc. Optic nerve injury often produces a central scotoma, with field loss in the macular region. A junctional scotoma with superior quadrantopia in one eye and an optic nerve defect in the other indicates a lesion at the junction of optic nerve with chiasm. This is seen because a few fibers from one optic nerve dip forward into the nerve of the opposite eye and may be compressed; it is highly suggestive of a suprasellar tumor.

A bitemporal defect is a field loss in both temporal regions. Chiasmal lesions affect nasal fibers from both eyes as they cross centrally and thus may cause bitemporal defects. Homonymous hemianopic defects are produced by lesions of the optic tract. The more congruous (or similar) the defects are in the two eyes, the more posterior the lesions are in the optic tracts. If there is macular sparing, the lesion is most likely in the occipital lobe. If the defect is less clear when tested with large objects than with small, the causative lesion is more likely to be compressive than vascular.

Homonymous defects involve the same portion of both visual fields. Homonymous quadrantopic defects involve part of the optic radiations. A lesion in Meyer's loop around the temporal horn will produce a "pie-in-the-sky" defect or "superior" quandrantopia. In all of these the brain lesion is on the opposite side from the field defect.

Oculomotor (III), Trochlear (IV), and Abducens (VI) Nerves

Lesions in these nerves produce ocular movement and pupillary defects. The triad of incomplete eye movements, pupil asymmetry and ptosis suggests a third nerve lesion; if there is no pupil asymmetry, diabetes is a likely cause. Ptosis plus pupillary dilation (from compression of the parasympathetic fibers that run in III) suggests a mass such as an internal carotid aneurysm, compressing the third nerve in the tentorial notch.

Failure of abduction in one eye implies a sixth nerve lesion. This may be spontaneous and completely recoverable, but may also represent increased intracranial pressure as the sixth nerve is very sensitive to compressive forces. Double vision with most difficulty on looking down to read suggests a fourth nerve lesion; it usually occurs with atherosclerosis or trauma. A very specific syndrome in which one eye fails to adduct on looking to one side but can do so on convergence is called an internuclear ophthalmoplegia (INO); there may be nystagmus of the abducting eye as well. It is patho-

second test to distinguish conductive from sensorineural loss is the Weber test. For this, a vibrating tuning fork is placed at the center of the forehead: with conductive loss from middle ear disease, the sound will be heard in the deaf ear better; with sensorineural loss it will be louder in the good ear.

The glossopharyngeal nerve (IX) is tested by noting symmetry of uvula movement and sensation in the pharynx (gag reflex). The accessory nerve (XI) is tested by asking the patient to turn his or her chin against the examiner's hand; a defective left nerve will make turning to the right weak.

The hypoglossal (XII) nerve is tested by evaluating the tongue for midline position and fasciculations. With a weak left XII nerve the tongue will deviate to the left on extension.

Motor testing begins with examination of muscle groups for atrophy, involuntary movements, or fasciculations (small rippling under the skin). Each muscle group listed in Table 1.1 should be tested by the corresponding maneuvers. Strength is graded from 0 to 5 as follows: 0- no contraction, 1- trace contraction, 2- movement that does not overcome gravity, 3- active movement against gravity, 4- active movement against resistance, 5- full strength. Tone is also estimated to be normal, increased, or decreased.

Table 1.1. Muscle Function and Innervation

Muscle	Movement	Major Root	Nerve
deltoid	arm elevation	C5	axillary
biceps	forearm flexion	C6	musculocutaneous
triceps	forearm extension	C7	radial
extensor carpi ulnaris	wrist extension	C7	posterior interosseous
opponens pollicus	thumb opposition	C8	median
finger flexors (pip joint)	grasp	C8	median
dorsal interossei	spreading fingers	T1	ulnar
iliopsoas	hip flexion	L2	femoral
quadriceps	leg extension	L3	femoral
tibialis anterior	foot dorsiflexion	L5	deep peroneal
extensor hallicus	great toe dorsiflexion	L5	deep peroneal
gluteus maximus	hip extension	L5	inferior gluteal
hamstrings	leg flexion	S1	sciatic
gastrocnemius	foot plantar flexion	S1	tibial nerve

darkened room. The optic disc itself is examined for pallor or blurring of the disc margins, the retina for hemorrhage or exudates, and the retinal vessels for venous pulsations, narrowing or atherosclerosis. A long-distance (20 feet) eye chart should be used for acuity; a near-vision card is a less sensitive test. The visual fields are named temporal (to the side) and nasal (toward the nose) as the patient sees them. To test the fields, a 5-mm white object such as a pinhead is gradually brought into the upper or lower nasal or temporal field of one eye at a time.

The oculomotor, trochlear, and abducens nerves (III, IV, VI) are tested together by examining convergence (looking at one's nose), vertical and lateral eye movements, coordination of eye movements, lid droop, and pupillary size and reactivity. These functions reflect not only the cranial nerves but also the brainstem regions that contain their nuclei and the tracts that connect and influence them.

The trigeminal (V) nerve has both sensory and motor functions and three divisions. Pin and light touch should be tested over the forehead (V1), cheek (V2), and chin (V3); the corneal reflex tests V1 and the nostril tickle V2. Deviation of the jaw to either side tests the motor division of the trigeminal nerve: the motor root of the right trigeminal nerve supplies the right masseter muscle, making deviation of jaw to the left difficult.

Functions of the facial nerve (VII) include facial motion, taste in the anterior two-thirds of the tongue, salivation, tearing, sensation of the inner ear and tonsils, and stapedius muscle innervation. The nerve is tested by asking the patient to smile, frown, and pucker, and by testing perception of salt and sugar on the anterior tongue. An enlarged palpebral fissure can be a subtle sign of facial muscle weakness.

Testing of the auditory nerve (VIII) begins by making certain that the ear canals are free of wax, then whispering in one ear while scratching on a card held beside the other to block its hearing. If a whisper cannot be heard 12 inches from the ear, there is hearing loss. The next step is to assess whether the loss is conductive or neural; for this, a 512 cps tuning fork is held against the mastoid process and then held up to the ear after the patient has stopped hearing it. If the patient can hear the fork again, this is a normal or "positive" Rinné (air conduction is better than bone conduction). If there is conductive hearing loss, the fork will still not be heard. A

Reflexes to be tested include jaw jerk (V3), biceps (C5–6), triceps (C7), knee jerk (L3–4), ankle jerk (S1), abdominal (T10, T12), and cremasteric reflexes (S2–3). They should be the same on either side. An important pathological reflex to be tested is the Babinski sign, an extension of the great toe with fanning of the other toes on stroking the foot with a pointed object such as a key. A positive response indicates a lesion in the corticospinal tract. However, the sign is not easy to interpret in some cases.

Tests of lateral *cerebellar function* include finger-nose-finger (the ability to touch the examiner's finger and then one's own nose) and heel-knee-shin (the ability to run the heel of one foot along the shin). *Gait* should be specifically tested in every patient, looking for unsteadiness, limping, leg weakness, and the ability to walk a straight line.

Testing *sensation* is often the most difficult part of the examination to perform accurately, especially avoiding suggestions to the patient. There are two types of sensory testing—primary and cortical. For primary sensory function, vibration is tested with a 128 or 256 cps tuning fork on bony prominences, while joint position sense is tested with 5-mm movements of the digit (with care not to press on the top or bottom of the toe or finger). Light touch is best assessed with a tissue wisp, comparing sides. Pain testing is done with a pin, comparing sides; it should not be done with a hypodermic needle, as this punctures the skin very readily.

Cortical sensory testing involves more complex stimuli. Stereognostic testing is done by placing objects in the patient's palm or drawing numbers in the palm (graphesthesia testing), which the patient has to identify with closed eyes. Two-point discrimination is tested by touching the skin simultaneously with objects a certain distance apart. Double simultaneous stimulation is carried out by touching both sides of the body or limb at once. These procedures test parietal lobe function.

Often during the history and examination the surgeon will be able to form a satisfactory idea of *mental status;* however, several aspects of mental status should be tested explicitly. Speech is assessed by listening to spontaneous speech and by testing for repetition, naming, reading, writing, and copying. Manipulative ability or praxis should be tested by observing the patient use scissors or matches, or button a coat. Memory is tested first by asking several questions regarding common knowledge, then by asking the patient to remember three words and asking him or her to repeat them after a period of distraction. If defects are found, more detailed testing should be done as described in specialty texts.

The Neurological Examination in Infants and Young Children

In infants, the neurological examination is based on the stages of normal development. Several reflexes found in a newborn should not persist beyond three months: these include the sucking reflex, a pursing of the lips when a lip is stroked; the grasp reflex, an involuntary gripping of the fingers placed in the palm; and the Moro reflex, a rapid abduction of the arms when the child is suddenly lowered while being held supine. The plantar reflex may remain normally extensor to age 2 or 3 years. Limb tone is an important aspect of the motor examination, providing clues about possible neurologic abnormalities.

Some important landmarks in development are as follows: a moving object is followed with the eyes at 12 weeks, sitting with support is possible at 24 weeks, and crawling and standing should be possible at 40 weeks. Walking and speaking have quite variable ages of onset, but are present in 90 percent of children by 14 and 13 months, respectively.

Vision can be tested in an infant by using a moving object or light, and hearing by observing the response to a loud noise. The head circumference can be plotted accurately on a percentile chart, but in general a 3-month child should have a head circumference of 38–43 cm, a 6-month child 41–46 cm, a 12-month child 44–49 cm, and a 24-month child 46–52 cm.

Abnormalities in the Neurological Examination

Cranial Nerves

Olfactory (I)

Inability to smell (*anosmia*) may result from local disease in the nose, such as chronic nasal infection, polyps, or tumor. The most common cause, however, is an old injury of the olfactory tract. A subfrontal meningioma or another tumor compressing the olfactory tract may also cause anosmia.

Optic (II)

The optic nerve may demonstrate abnormalities on funduscopic examination, in visual acuity, or in visual field. On funduscopic examination, the normal optic disc is pink and well-demarcated with visible venous pulsations. The most important fundoscopic abnormality to recognize is papilledema—swelling of the optic nerve head that results from blockage to axoplasmic flow. The edges of the entire disc become indistinct. Central veins become engorged and nonpulsatile, and hemorrhages may develop as well as exudates in the retina. Papilledema is caused by increased intracranial pressure or arterial hypertension. There is usually no visual acuity loss except an enlarged blind spot. This feature differentiates it from optic neuritis, in which visual loss from a central scotoma may be severe. It often takes expert help to make the differential diagnosis between true papilledema and such conditions as optic drusen and pseudopapilledema. If there is doubt, consult a neuro-ophthalmologist. Untreated papilledema can progress to optic atrophy and blindness.

In *optic atrophy* the disc is pale and sharp; this always represents disease of the optic nerve or chiasm. Multiple sclerosis with optic neuritis, primary optic nerve tumors such as meningiomas or gliomas, tumors directly compressing the optic nerve or chiasm such as pituitary tumors or suprasellar meningiomas, central retinal artery occlusion, old glaucoma or papilledema, methyl alcohol intoxication, and some drugs can cause optic atrophy. In children, cerebromacular degeneration is also a possible cause.

Numerous problems may lead to *loss of visual acuity,* including corneal, lenticular, and retinal disorders and intracranial disease. Acuity loss from intracranial disease is usually accompanied by a visual field defect. Loss of acuity in one eye means disease of the optic nerve or orbit. A bitemporal loss suggests chiasmal compression, usually from a pituitary tumor.

Visual field testing is done either by moving spherical objects such as the head of a pin into view or by diminishing the brightness of lights kept stationary. Visual field evaluation can provide valuable information about diseases of the optic nerve and tracts. In reading fields, the middle of the field as displayed is perpendicular to the macula; the temporal field (70°) is wider than nasal (50°), and fields are presented as though you were looking at them; field deficits are described as nasal or temoral and upper or lower.

Three field patterns imply retinal disease: an arcuate defect from central retinal artery ischemia, an inferior hemianopia in one eye suggesting a vascular lesion, and an enlarged blind spot caused by an enlarged optic disc. Optic nerve injury often produces a central scotoma, with field loss in the macular region. A junctional scotoma with superior quadrantopia in one eye and an optic nerve defect in the other indicates a lesion at the junction of optic nerve with chiasm. This is seen because a few fibers from one optic nerve dip forward into the nerve of the opposite eye and may be compressed; it is highly suggestive of a suprasellar tumor.

A bitemporal defect is a field loss in both temporal regions. Chiasmal lesions affect nasal fibers from both eyes as they cross centrally and thus may cause bitemporal defects. Homonymous hemianopic defects are produced by lesions of the optic tract. The more congruous (or similar) the defects are in the two eyes, the more posterior the lesions are in the optic tracts. If there is macular sparing, the lesion is most likely in the occipital lobe. If the defect is less clear when tested with large objects than with small, the causative lesion is more likely to be compressive than vascular.

Homonymous defects involve the same portion of both visual fields. Homonymous quadrantopic defects involve part of the optic radiations. A lesion in Meyer's loop around the temporal horn will produce a "pie-in-the-sky" defect or "superior" quandrantopia. In all of these the brain lesion is on the opposite side from the field defect.

Oculomotor (III), Trochlear (IV), and Abducens (VI) Nerves

Lesions in these nerves produce ocular movement and pupillary defects. The triad of incomplete eye movements, pupil asymmetry and ptosis suggests a third nerve lesion; if there is no pupil asymmetry, diabetes is a likely cause. Ptosis plus pupillary dilation (from compression of the parasympathetic fibers that run in III) suggests a mass such as an internal carotid aneurysm, compressing the third nerve in the tentorial notch.

Failure of abduction in one eye implies a sixth nerve lesion. This may be spontaneous and completely recoverable, but may also represent increased intracranial pressure as the sixth nerve is very sensitive to compressive forces. Double vision with most difficulty on looking down to read suggests a fourth nerve lesion; it usually occurs with atherosclerosis or trauma. A very specific syndrome in which one eye fails to adduct on looking to one side but can do so on convergence is called an internuclear ophthalmoplegia (INO); there may be nystagmus of the abducting eye as well. It is pathognomonic of a brain stem lesion in the medial longitudinal fasciculus and is usually caused by multiple sclerosis or, rarely, from stroke.

Abnormalities of conjugate gaze are helpful in localizing a disease process. Failure of conjugate upgaze suggests a lesion in the midbrain collicular plate or increased intracranial pressure. Failure or weakness of conjugate gaze to one side can result from a lesion in the frontal or parieto-occipital lobe on the same side as the weakness, or to pontine gaze centers on the opposite side. Frontal and parietal regions can be distinguished by the fact that parietal visual centers control pursuit movements (following an object) and frontal centers saccadic movement (looking to the left or right).

The evaluation of *diplopia* may be difficult if there are no obvious III, IV, or VI lesions. One helpful rule is that the widest separation of images occurs in the axis of movement of the weak muscle; a second is that monocular diplopia (diplopia with one eye closed) results from disease of the lens or globe, not from extraocular muscle weakness.

Nystagmus, involuntary eye jerkiness with both fast and slow components, may be a sign of alcohol or barbituate intoxication; a small amount is normal. By convention, the direction of the fast component is used to report its orientation. It is always a sign of brainstem or cerebellar dysfunction if abnormal in degree. Special testing such as electronystagmography can help establish its cause and extent.

The *pupils* are tested to evaluate autonomic as well as brain stem function. Anisocoria or difference in pupil diameter is present in 15 percent of the population; this normal variation is called "physiological anisocoria." The diagnosis of physiological anisocoria is established by moving from a light to a dark room and noting that the pupillary difference remains the same. If the anisocoria increases in the dark, the small pupil is the abnormal one, and the pupillary dilator function has failed. If the anisocoria increases in the light, the large pupil is the abnormal one, with pupillary sphincter failure. The *Marcus-Gunn phenomenon* is a very sensitive indicator of retinal or optic nerve disease (afferent pupillary defect). Testing is done by moving a bright light source from the good eye to the bad one. The Marcus-Gunn phenomenon is defined as dilation of the pupil when light is shone directly into the affected eye after it has been shone into the unaffected one. It implies an optic nerve or retinal defect and is not a measure of visual acuity. The *Argyll-Robertson* pupil is small and does not react to light but does react to accommodation. It is formally defined as a miotic irregular pupil in a seeing eye that has no reaction to light, some reaction to accommodation, and dilates poorly to eye drops. It is important because it is pathognomic of syphilis. A more common finding, however, is so-called *light-near dissociation,* in which the reaction to light is not as good as that to accommodation. This more common pupillary abnormality can be associated with syphilis, diabetes, lesions of the periaqueductal gray, tectal compression from a pineal tumor, Adie's tonic pupil, and aberrant third nerve regeneration.

A pupil that does not appear to react to light or accommodation is usually a case of *Adie's tonic pupil.* It is of importance in neurosurgery because it may be mistaken for the pupil of a third nerve compressive lesion (see below). It usually occurs in women unilaterally or bilaterally and is accompanied by a loss of knee and ankle jerks. To light, the pupil reacts slowly and has an even slower but definite constriction to accommodation. It then dilates slowly. It is probably caused by a loss of parasympathetic fibers from the ciliary ganglion with aberrant regeneration and subsequent inadequacy of dilator function. The definitive diagnosis is made by demonstrating denervation hypersensitivity with a weak solution of 2–5 percent mecholyl that causes constriction in this pupil but not in a normal pupil.

The dilated pupil unresponsive to light or accommodation that is so feared by neurosurgeons is called *Hutchinson's pupil.* It signifies compression of the oculomotor nerve by an intracranial mass and means incipient or already progressive uncal herniation. It can occur bilaterally during seizures.

If evaluation has shown a small pupil unable to dilate, *Horner's syndrome* is likely. Ptosis, apparent enophthalmos, and possibly decreased sweating accompany the small pupil. Ten percent cocaine should dilate a normal pupil by norepinephrine release; it will not do so in Horner's and will therefore establish a diagnosis. Lesions anywhere in the sympathetic chain can produce Horner's syndrome. Twenty percent of patients with Horner's syndrome harbor a malignant lesion, often of the paranasal sinuses; 20 percent have no apparent cause. Causes at the level of the brain stem or first-order neuron of the sympathetic system include brain stem stroke, syringomyelia, syringobulbia, brain stem or cervical cord tumor, and neurosyphilis. Second-order neurons (in the cervical sympathetic chain) may be affected by cervical surgery or trauma, a pancoast tumor, or cervical rib. Third order neurons (from superior cervical ganglion along the carotid sheath) may be damaged by angiomas, carotid surgery, otitis media, cholesteatomas, or skull fracture.

Trigeminal (V)

The trigeminal nerve is rarely defective except in tumors of the cerebellopontine angle. If facial pain is accompanied by sensory or motor defects referable to this nerve, trigeminal neuralgia is an unlikely diagnosis.

Facial (VII)

Facial nerve dysfunction offers an opportunity for very selective anatomical diagnosis as to the site of dysfunction; neurology texts provide details. Facial weakness most often results from Bell's palsy but may also reflect an acoustic neuroma. If the weakness stems from a tumor, hearing loss will invariably accompany it.

Acoustic and Vestibular (VIII)

The most common neurosurgical cause of hearing loss is a vestibular schwannoma (also called acoustic neuroma). In any adult with sensorineural hearing loss a neuroma should be considered, even though it is not the most common cause of hearing loss.

Glossopharyngeal (IX), Vagus (X), Accessory (XI), and Hypoglossal (XII)

These nerves may be damaged by tumors of the base of the brain or by basilar artery thrombosis. The glossopharyngeal nerve regulates sensation of the soft palate, vagus the heart rate, accessory the power of ipsilateral sternomastoid, and hypoglossal tongue protrusion. Glossopharyngeal dysfunction produces a poor gag reflex and the palate does not elevate symmetrically. Loss of the right hypoglossal nerve causes tongue deviation to the right on protrusion.

Cortical Signs and Symptoms

Aphasia

Aphasia is best defined as a disorder of language with a defect in either the production or comprehension of vocabulary or syntax. One classification proposed by Geschwind divides aphasia into nonfluent and fluent types. *Nonfluent* (Broca's) aphasia is characterized by sparse, poorly articulated speech; the patient is usually aware of the difficulty. The anatomical correlate is injury to Broca's area in the third frontal gyrus; the main problem is difficulty with speech output. *Fluent* aphasia implies a defect in language comprehension and is classified according to the patient's ability to understand spoken language and to repeat phrases. *Wernicke's* aphasia involves impairment of both comprehension and repetition. The patient is unaware of the deficit and has normal melody of speech but utters many wrong words. This is associated with injury to the posterior part of the superior temporal gyrus of the dominant hemisphere and often has few associated neurological signs. In *conduction* aphasia, comprehension is intact but repetition is poor. Literal paraphasias (words sounding the same as the correct word but often making no sense) are characteristic of conduction aphasia. This syndrome involves disruption of the arcuate fasciculus connecting Wernicke's and Broca's areas. *Anomic* aphasia is a fluent aphasia with both comprehension and repetition intact. Circumlocutions (phrases like "it's the thing that you do when you are . . .") and verbal paraphasias characterize this speech. Naming is especially impaired and writing is always defective. Anomic aphasia has little localizing value as it can occur with increased intracranial pressure, drug intoxication, and other diffuse processes such as Alzheimer's disease and head injury. When it is due to focal disease it implies a lesion at or below the angular gyrus. A final common aphasic syndrome is *global aphasia:* nonfluent speech with impairment of both comprehension and repetition. This is seen with strokes in the middle cerebral artery distribution.

In examining speech, problems with articulation, tone production, or dysarthria may confuse the evaluation. Dysarthria can arise from lower cranial nerve (IX, X, XI) or bilateral corticobulbar tract damage. Cerebellar disorders may produce scanning speech with improper accentuation of syllables because of an incoordination between respiratory and articular efforts. Lisping and stuttering, two common speech disorders, do not have localizing value. Mutism from upper brain stem damage involves minimal speech function but is easy to identify by its other manifestations, cranial nerve and limb weakness.

Cortical Sensory Defects

Parietal cortical lesions cause disturbances in discriminatory sensation, which may include astereognosis (inability to understand the form and nature of objects by touch), abarognosis (poor recognition of weight), autopagnosia or somatoparagnosia (inability to identify or orient the body, or relation of individual parts), anosognosia (ignorance of the existence of disease), and sensory inattention (diagnosed as loss of the ability to perceive sensation on one side of the body when identical areas on both sides are stimulated). In general, parietal defects are characterized by a loss of the ability to recognize the meaning of stimuli rather than a loss in sensory reception itself. Gerstmann's syndrome, one constellation of dominant parietal lobe defects, comprises loss of awareness of position and identity of body parts, disorientation for right and left, inability to write (agraphia), inability to calculate (acalculia), and inability to recognize, name, and select individual fingers when looking at the hands.

Cortical Visual Field Defects

Visual field defects were discussed above. Several implicate the cortical pathways specifically. Congruous homonymous visual field defects indicate an occipital cortical lesion or a lesion in the pathways between the geniculate body and the cortex. Cortical blindness follows bilateral occipital lesions and is characterized by visual loss with intact pupillary reactions; the patient may not be aware of the visual defect. With damage farther forward in the occipital lobe, disturbance of space perception, inability to understand what one is seeing (visual agnosia), inability to read (alexia), loss of visual memory, denial of blindness, and loss of following and reflex movements of the eyes are characteristic.

Quadrantopias suggest an optic radiation lesion. A lower quadrantopia implies damage to fibers radiating through the parietal lobe and terminating on the upper lip of the calcarine fissure; an upper quadrantopia signifies involvement of fibers radiating in the temporal lobe and around the lateral ventricles.

Frontal Lobe Disorders

Symptoms of frontal lobe dysfunction include disinhibition, difficulty dealing with new material, inattention, emotional instability, irritability, and facetiousness.

Other Cortical Syndromes

The *Foster-Kennedy syndrome* is primary optic nerve atrophy on the side of the lesion together with concomitant papilledema in the opposite eye. It localizes a lesion to the anterior cranial fossa on the side of the atrophic optic nerve and may be caused by tumor, abscess, vascular abnormality, or local arachnoiditis over the atrophic optic nerve.

The *parasagittal lesion syndrome* includes weakness in the legs, focal motor or sensory seizures, incontinence of urine or feces, and mental changes or frontal lobe syndromes. It may mimic a spinal cord lesion because both legs are involved; the syndrome can be distinguished from spinal cord disease by the presence of seizures and mental changes and the asymmetry and incompleteness of leg weakness.

Parasellar lesions produce endocrine dysfunction that may lead to diabetes insipidus, visual loss especially of bitemporal type, alterations in sleep and appetitite, loss of temperature regulation suggesting hypothalamic dysfunction, and increased intracranial pressure.

Superior sagittal sinus occlusion can produce increased intracranial pressure, seizures, engorgement of scalp veins, and spastic paralysis.

Cavernous sinus syndromes include proptosis, chemosis, papilledema, dilated retinal veins and retinal hemorrhage, paralysis of the third, fourth, and sixth nerves as well as the first and second division of the fifth cranial nerve, pain in the eye, and normal or slightly impaired vision. They may be caused by a carotid aneurysm, a cavernous sinus fistula, a tumor in the sinus, or sinus thrombosis. Occlusion of the lateral sinuses may simply produce increased intracranial pressure.

Brain Stem Syndromes and Signs

Two kinds of deficit invariably implicate the brain stem: specific eye movement deficits as described above, and so-called "crossed paralyses" or alternating hemiplegia. In crossed paralyses a patient has sensory or motor deficits involving the cranial nerves on the side of the lesion and the arm or leg on the opposite side because the lesion occurs above the decussation of the medial lemniscus or corticospinal tract. Figure 1.1 illustrates the brainstem in longitudinal section.

When one is evaluating cranial nerve and motor findings, several brain stem syndromes of historical interest should be considered because they are important in establishing the precise location

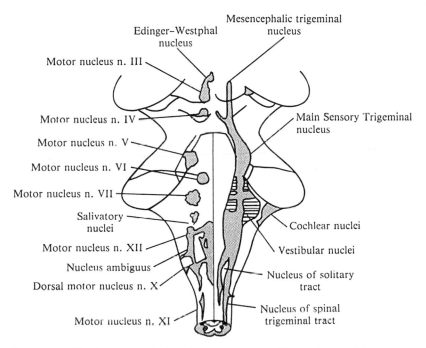

Figure 1.1. The brainstem in longitudinal section. The major nuclei are demonstrated.

of an infarct or other pathological process (see Table 1.2). In general these are vascular syndromes of most interest to the neurologist. There are also compressive lesions of the cranial nerves outside the brain stem; the syndrome of the cerebellopontine angle tumor and Vernet's syndrome of lower cranial nerve dysfunction are especially important to the neurosurgeon (Table 1.3). It should be noted that the sixth nerve is notoriously unreliable as an indicator of brain stem localization in that a sixth nerve palsy alone or with papilledema does not mean the lesion is anywhere near the sixth nerve. The dysfunction can be caused by stretching of the nerve as a result of generalized brain swelling.

Spinal Cord and Cauda Equina Syndromes

A distinction can be made between an upper motor neuron lesion, in which there is increased tone of an extremity and hyperactive

Table 1.2. Selected Brainstem Syndromes

Name	Structures	Signs	Usual Cause
Midbrain			
Weber	III nucleus, corticospinal tract	oculomotor palsy, contralateral hemiplegia	brain stem infarct
Benedict	III nucleus, corticospinal tract, cerebral peduncle	oculomotor palsy, crossed cerebellar ataxia and hemiplegia, tremor	brain stem infarct
Parinaud's	dorsal midbrain	upward gaze defective	pineal region tumor
Pons			
Millard-Guber	VI, VII, corticospinal tract	VI, VII palsy, ` contralateral hemiplegia	brain stem infarct
Medulla			
Wallenberg	VI, IX, X, XI, lateral spinothalamic, spinocerebellar tract, sympathetic fibers	ipsilateral VI, IX, X, XI palsy, Horner syndrome, cerebellar ataxia	occlusion of vertebral or posterior inferior artery

reflexes below the lesion, and a lower motor neuron lesion, in which there is flaccidity and areflexia at the level of the lesion. The upper motor neuron pattern is characteristic of cortical, brainstem, or spinal cord injury. Figure 1.2 is a cross section of the spinal cord and the major tracts.

Several features point to localization of a lesion in the spinal cord: bilaterally symmetrical sensory loss, flaccid weakness in one spinal cord segment with spastic weakness in limbs below that segment, and impairment of anal and urethral sphincter activity.

Several syndromes of spinal cord and cauda equina function are important for the neurosurgeon. The *lateral cauda equina syndrome* involves anterior thigh pain, quadriceps wasting, weakness of foot inversion, and an absent knee jerk; its most likely cause is a neurofibroma or other nerve root tumor. The *central cauda syndrome* is identical to the symptoms of a conus medullaris lesion with rectal

Table 1.3. Syndromes of Multiple Cranial Nerves in the Periphery

Name	Site Involved	Nerves	Usual Cause
Foix	sphenoid fissure	III, IV, V, VI	sphenoid tumors, aneurysms
Tolosa-Hunt	lateral wall of cavernous sinus	III, IV, V, VI	cavernous sinus aneurysm or thrombosis, invasive parasellar tumor; occasionally benign, and responds to steroids
Gradenigo	petrous apex	V, VI	petrous bone tumor or inflammation
Vernet	jugular foramen	IX, X, XI	tumor or aneurysm
Collet-Sicard	posterolateral condylar space	IX, X, XI, XII	parotid or carotid tumor, lymphoma
Villaret	posterolateral condylar space	Collet-Sicard and Horner's	same as Collet-Sicard but extending outside skull
Tapia	retroparotid space	X, XI, XII	parotid tumors

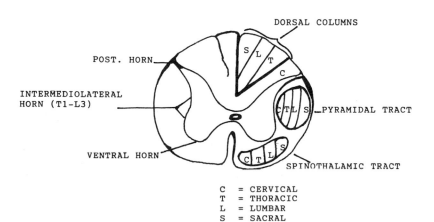

DORSAL COLUMNS

POST. HORN

INTERMEDIOLATERAL HORN (T1-L3)

VENTRAL HORN

PYRAMIDAL TRACT

SPINOTHALAMIC TRACT

C = CERVICAL
T = THORACIC
L = LUMBAR
S = SACRAL

Figure 1.2. Cross section of the spinal cord.

and genital pain, urinary disturbance, and paucity of findings unless perianal sensation is tested. An ependymoma, dermoid tumor, or lipoma of the terminal cord is the usual cause. Finally there is a syndrome of pain stemming from L5, S1, S2, or S3 roots, usually caused by extradural compression of roots by a ruptured intervertebral disc, chordoma, metastatic disease, leukemia, or seeding from CNS tumors.

An important syndrome involving the cord itself is the so-called "complete" syndrome, a total loss of sensory, motor, and autonomic function below a specific spinal cord level. There is initially a period of shock with flaccid total paralysis of all musculature and all reflexes, complete loss of cutaneous sensation, and transient urinary and fecal retention. Vasomotor instability is common and may be accompanied by bilateral Horner's syndrome when lesions are above T1. Over a period of 1 to 6 weeks spinal reflexes return, with clonus and the appearance of the Babinski sign. Flexor spasms and mass reflexes with profuse sweating and flushing may develop in response to cutaneous or other stimulation, and extensor spasms occur.

Brown-Sequard syndrome is homolateral upper motor neuron paralysis, vasomotor paralysis, and position and vibratory loss below the level of the lesion with contralateral loss of pain and temperature sensation. Practically speaking, homolateral spastic weakness with a contralateral sensory loss is the most important symptom; there may be varying partial loss. Any process encroaching asymmetrically on the spinal cord may produce this syndrome.

The *anterior spinal artery syndrome* is characterized by bilateral motor paralysis and cutaneous sensory loss below the affected level with sparing of position and vibratory sensation. It can be caused by infarction of the anterior spinal artery, but also is important to recognize after trauma as it may mean disc rupture.

The *syringomyelia syndrome* is characterized by dissociation of pain and temperature sensation loss, with loss of pinprick sensation on one side and temperature loss on the other. There may also be a segmental sensory loss.

The *central cord syndrome* is characterized by weakness of the hands more than the legs, mild bladder incontinence, and gait difficulty. It is a result of central cord injury in the cervical region and is a common finding after cervical trauma in the elderly.

Peripheral Nerve Symptoms and Signs

The peripheral nerves are formed by complex combinations of spinal roots in the cervical and lumbosacral plexus. The neurosurgeon should be familiar with this organizational pattern, which is discussed in Chapter 10. The nerves are mixed nerves containing both motor and sensory fibers. Characteristic abnormalities are weakness with sensory loss of all modalities, fasciculations, retention of sphincter tone, and hyporeflexia (Table 1.4).

Skeletal Muscle Symptoms and Signs

Muscle disorders are most important in neurosurgery as mimickers of spinal cord or peripheral nervous system lesions. They can generally be identified by the following features: motor loss is flaccid and especially prominent in muscles of the trunk and proximal limbs rather than distally; cutaneous reflexes are preserved and there are no pathological reflexes such as Babinski or Hoffman signs; sensation and sphincter control are preserved.

A Comment on Etiological Diagnosis

This chapter has dealt primarily with anatomical diagnosis—the localization of neurologic findings. The rest of this book is mainly about etiological diagnosis—the cause of particular neurological symptoms. Here a few words may be appropriate on the temporal pattern of different types of disorders, related to their cause. *Congenital disorders* tend to be established and present from birth. *Neoplasms* usually have gradual onset, although a seizure or hemorrhage caused by a trauma may lead to a strokelike syndrome. *Vascular diseases* usually have sudden onset, progression to maximal deficit in minutes to hours, plateau, and then improvement. *Demyelinating diseases* differ from vascular disease in the progressive accumulation of deficits. Multiple sclerosis, acute encephalomyelitis, and diffuse cerebral sclerosis are important to neurosurgeons because they can mimic brain tumors. *Degenerative diseases* are gradual in onset, progressive for many years, and often involve several systems. *Metabolic diseases* may mimic tumors or degenerative

2

Radiological Diagnosis
in Neurosurgery

Some of the most significant advances relevant to neurosurgery in recent years have come from neuroradiology. Diagnoses of many diseases that were difficult years ago are now easily and accurately made with modern imaging techniques. In this chapter we will discuss the most common neuroradiologic studies available, as well as when they are most indicated.

Skull Films

With the increasing availability of CT and MRI, the plain skull film is ordered much less frequently. There are occasions, however, when it is not only a good screening study, but also provides valuable information to help make a diagnosis.

One of the most common current uses of skull films is to evaluate head injury. While useful in making the diagnosis of a skull fracture, skull films are less helpful than CT scanning in determining the extent of intracranial pathology. The use of skull films in the evaluation of trauma should be limited to defining the extent of depressed skull fractures and documenting the presence of foreign bodies. Skull films are also useful in showing congenital abnormalities due to craniosynostosis and in diagnosing lytic lesions. The radiologic characteristics of several skull lesions are summarized in Table 2.1.

Table 2.1. Skull Lesions

Diagnosis	X-Ray Characteristics
Eosinophic granuloma	Usually single lesion with irregular margins without any sclerosis
Multiple myeloma	Multiple punched out lesions with sharp borders
Epidermoid	Single lesion with a smooth sclerotic border of bone
Metastatic lesion(s)	Single or multiple lesions with or without sclerosis and poorly defined irregular margins
Hemangioma	"Sunburst" appearance of single sharp bordered lesion without sclerosis
Osteomyelitis	Single or multiple sclerotic lesions with irregular borders
Histiocytosis X	Multiple nonsclerotic lesions with well defined margins

Intracranial calcifications are another finding that may be significant on skull films. There may be normal calcifications (in pineal, petroclinoid ligament, choroid plexus, falx, tentorium, dural plaques, arachnoid granulations, habenula, basal ganglia, and dentate nucleus) and abnormal (aneurysms, AVMs, tumors, and phakomatoses).

Other important skull erosions include an enlarged internal auditory canal produced by acoustic neuromas; clivus erosion caused by large pituitary adenomas, chordomas, nasopharyngeal carcinomas, and metastatic tumors; and optic foramina enlargement caused by nerve sheath meningiomas or optic gliomas.

Spine Films

Plain spine X-rays are mostly used for the initial workup of spinal trauma and pain patients. Based on the results of these studies, a CT scan or MRI may then be obtained either to define an abnormality better or to look for one that the plain film is not able to demonstrate. Five lines are used to study alignment of the cervical spine: the anterior or soft tissue line; the anterior spinal line formed by the anterior margins of the vertebral bodies; the posterior spinal line; the spinal lamina line; and the spinous process line. In assessing the cervical spine film, one should also evaluate the vertebral bodies (look for fractures, displacements, or changes in height), the disc space, and the intervertebral foramina (look for narrowing). Figure 2.1 shows a lateral cervical spine X-ray and CT reconstruction of a fracture at the base of the dens.

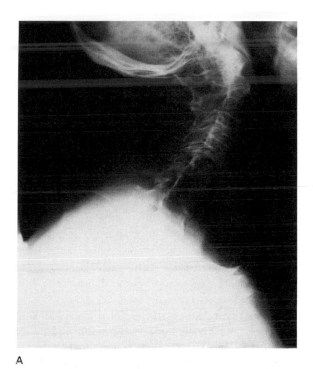

A

B

Figure 2.1. (A) Lateral cervical spine X-ray and (B) CT reconstruction of a fracture of the dens.

In suspected trauma of the cervical spine, the initial study should be a lateral cross table view with the neck immobilized. All seven cervical vertebrae as well as the top of the first thoracic vertebra should be seen; it may be necessary to place downward traction on the arms to be able to see C7 and T1. A swimmer's view is another possible way to visualize C7. A complete set of anteroposterior, oblique, and odontoid views should then be obtained. If there is neck tenderness, but no abnormality on the standard X-ray views, flexion and extension views should be performed to rule out ligamentous injury leading to instability without fracture. These flexion-extension views should only be done in the presence of a physician who is capable of assessing the patient's neurologic status during movement of the spine. Any increased pain, numbness, "electric shocks," or other symptoms related to the neck movement mandate immediate cessation of that movement and return to the neutral position.

Thoracic spine fractures occur in 20 percent of the spine fractures seen in patients with multiple trauma. They are most common in the mid-thoracic area. The most frequent findings are compression fractures with widening of the body and loss of height. Alignment should also be assessed.

Suspected trauma to the lumbar spine is evaluated in a similar way with AP, lateral, and, if indicated, oblique views. Again, it is important to view the vertebral body (looking for alignment, loss of height, obvious fracture), the disc space, the soft tissue, and the sacrum.

Vertebral osteomyelitis late in its course shows destructive erosion of contiguous vertebral bodies with sclerosis. There may be a paravertebral mass, and, in tuberculosis, scalloping of the anterior vertebral body. With infection, the disc space is the first structure to be destroyed. This differentiates a destructive lesion from tumor in which the disc space is generally spared. Malignant tumors that are metastatic to vertebral bodies present with pain or neurologic disability. Erosion of one pedicle, the winking owl sign, is suggestive of this process.

Myelography

As MRI and CT scanning have become more common, the number of myelograms performed has decreased dramatically. In some cases with spinal instrumentation, metal artifact on CT or MRI

Table 2.2. Differential Diagnosis of Spinal Canal Lesions

Location	Radiologic Appearance	Possible Lesions
Extradural	displaced thecal sac in one view and possible widening in another view: "feathered" margin	hematoma herniated disk bone spur metastatic lesion lymphoma neurofibroma epidural abscess
Intradural Extramedullary	displacement of the contrast column laterally and deviation of cord—smooth margin	neurofibroma meningioma lipoma drop metastasis dermoid(s)
Intradural Intramedullary	expansion of spinal cord and thinning of contrast column— tapered margin	astrocytoma ependymoma dermoid syringomyelia hematoma

makes myelography the only useful study, however. It consists of placing a contrast agent into the subarachnoid space, usually in the lumbar area (but the dye can also be placed through C2 puncture or cisternal puncture), and then taking multiple X-rays to demonstrate the flow of the contrast agent in the spinal canal and around nerve roots. Post-myelogram CT scans can also be done to define better any abnormalities demonstrated by the myelogram. Table 2.2 lists the differential diagnosis of some lesions seen on myelogram according to location.

Angiography

Angiography is another radiological study whose indications have changed with the introduction of CT and MRI scanning; however, there are still many cases where it can give information no other study can match. As MRI angiography becomes more advanced, there will probably be still further erosion of the indications for standard angiograms in the future.

The current indications for angiograms include evaluating subarachnoid hemorrhage, carotid or other vessel occlusive disease, vascular malformations, suspected aneurysms, vascular masses, ve-

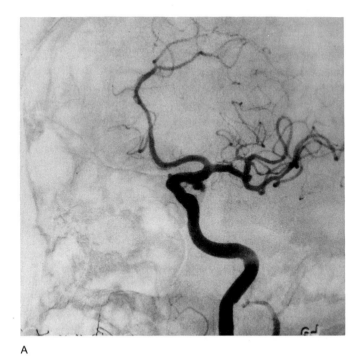

A

Figure 2.2. (A) AP and (B) lateral views of a cerebral arteriogram showing a posterior communicating artery aneurysm. This has the typical configuration of a so-called "berry" aneurysm.

nous sinuses, and arterial trauma. Some centers also perform invasive angiographically guided procedures such as coil occlusion of aneurysms and embolization of feeding vessels of vascular malformations and tumors. Figure 2.2 shows the arteriogram of a patient with a posterior communicating artery aneurysm.

Ultrasound

Ultrasound is used both diagnostically and intraoperatively to help localize lesions. In the antenatal period it is used to look for birth defects and in the postnatal period to evaluate intracerebral and intraventricular hemorrhage and hydrocephalus. It also serves as a noninvasive way to look at vascular lesions such as carotid stenosis or intracranial vasospasm. Currently, transcranial doppler ultraso-

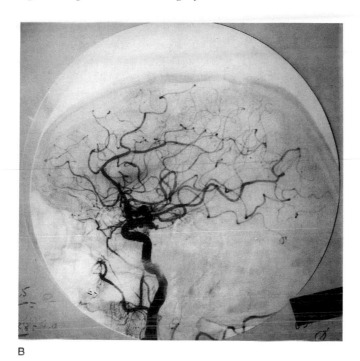

B

Figure 2.2. (continued)

nography is most useful in evaluating the progression of vasospasm following subarachnoid hemorrhage.

CT Scanning

Using computer analysis of photon absorption by different parts of the brain and skull, CT scanning can reveal a wide range of abnormalities noninvasively. Contrast agents are available to improve images of lesions that open the blood brain barrier or have an increased vascular supply. CT scanning evaluates the radiodensity of various structures. The most dense objects are the brightest (white) and the least dense objects the darkest (black).

In acute hematomas, a CT scan will show a white lesion, which is the clotted blood, against the gray background of the brain. An epidural hematoma is sharply defined against the skull with a bicon-vex (lenticular) appearance. The cranial sutures tend to either limit the extent of the epidural hematoma or affect its shape (Fig. 2.3). A subdural hematoma tends to diffuse along the surface of the brain, giving a semilunar (crescentic) appearance. In 3–4 weeks, a subdural hematoma will become isodense with the brain as it dissolves. Several weeks later, if not totally absorbed, the subdural hematoma may appear as a hypodense lesion, now called a chronic subdural hematoma. Figure 2.4 shows a chronic subdural hematoma with an acute component. Intraparenchymal hematomas appear as irregular, hyperintense, white lesions often with surrounding edema (hypo-

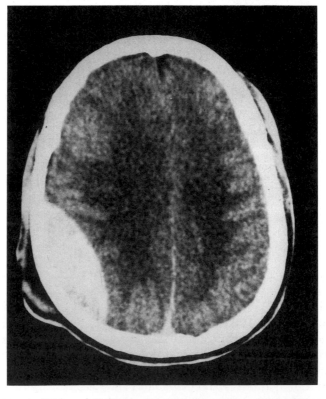

Figure 2.3. A CT scan of a right parietal epidural hematoma. The hematoma is sharply defined against the skull with a biconvex (lenticular) appearance. The cranial sutures limit the distribution of the blood.

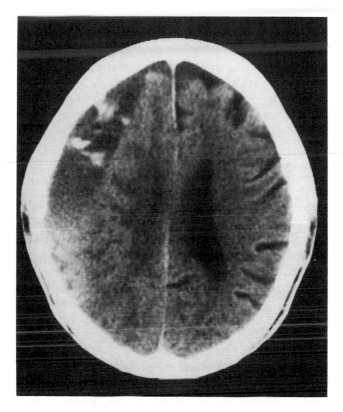

Figure 2.4. CT of a chronic subdural hematoma with an acute component. The chronic part is hypodense while the acute portion is hyperintense.

density) as time goes on. As they dissolve, the CT scan will show the density of the blood to decrease, often with increasing edema (hypodensity). Hematomas in the posterior fossa may be difficult to visualize because of the great amount of bone artifact present. Coronal views may help with this, as may an MRI, if needed. Figure 2.5 shows a left basal ganglia hypertensive hemorrhage that has extended into the ventricular system. Subarachnoid hemorrhage is seen on CT scan by the hyperdensity of the blood in the subarachnoid spaces and sometimes in the cortical sulci. There may be an associated communicating hydrocephalus. Brain contusions, revealed by a hyperintense spot in the brain substance, can also be

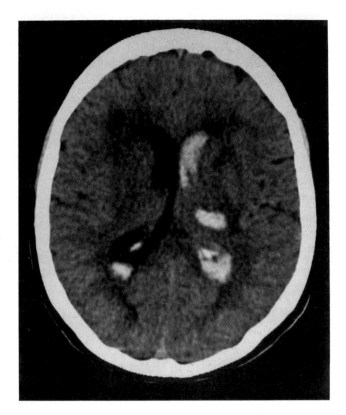

Figure 2.5. Intraparenchymal hematomas appear as irrregular
hyperintense white lesions often with surrounding edema. This CT shows
a left basal ganglia hypertensive hemorrhage that has extended into the
ventricular system.

detected. These tend to appear either directly at the site of trauma
(coup) or at a more distant site (contre-coup).

Hydrocephalus is revealed by increased ventricular size. Periventricular edema, bilateral symmetrical temporal horn enlargement, and ballooning or rounding of the frontal horns suggest obstructive hydrocephalus. Infarcts show as parenchymal lucency that
follows a vascular pattern. Dry infarcts are hypodense; wet infarcts
involve bleeding into the infarcted area and will therefore show hyperintense blood. Arachnoid cysts are smooth-walled masses with
CSF density. Epidermoids may have an even lower absorption value
than CSF.

Brain tumors generally appear as enhancing masses of varying internal consistency with edema. They may also have calcifications and can have significant mass effect. Glioblastomas are irregular enhancing masses with central necrosis (Fig. 2.6). Metastatic tumors may have an enhancing ring around them, as do abscesses. Both may produce edema and it may be hard to differentiate them without obtaining a tissue biopsy. Lymphomas appear as moderately uniform enhancing lesions that may not be seen on noncontrast studies.

Meningiomas generally enhance with contrast. They can be very large and may or may not have associated edema. Sometimes calcium is evident on the noncontrast CT. Meningiomas are usually dural based and brightly enhancing. Figure 2.7 shows the CT and MRI of a patient with a large meningioma. Vestibular schwannomas uniformly enhance and are present in the cerebellar pontine angle.

Vascular lesions that may be seen on CT include arteriovenous malformations, which are brightly enhancing. If the patient already has had a hemorrhage, there may be bright enhancement on contrast CT scan that is not present on the noncontrast study. Aneurysms may be seen on contrast CT if they are large enough, and the sections are thin enough through the area of the circle of Willis.

Multiple sclerosis plaques may appear as enhancing lesions or as small, focal, low-density white matter lesions.

CT scanning is also used in conjunction with stereotactic devices to help localize difficult-to-find or small lesions deep below the surface of the brain.

Magnetic Resonance Imaging

The addition of MRI to neurodiagnostic imaging over the past few years has enabled us to see pathology with much greater detail than has ever been possible noninvasively. It is proving to be as revolutionary as CT scanning in neurosurgery. It works by placing a strong magnetic field on the object to be scanned and then evaluating the change in certain fundamental properties of its atoms. Contrast agents can also be used to define certain lesions, as in CT scanning. Gadolineum is the most common paramagnetic contrast agent used today in MRI scanning.

In general, MRI shows more abnormalities than CT with a higher resolution and sensitivity. It is also possible to view the images in different planes with the data obtained, without the re-

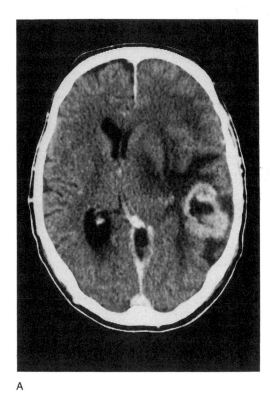

A

Figure 2.6. (A) CT and (B) MRI of a patient with glioblastoma multiforme.

scanning and repositioning that would be needed with CT. Standard
images include axial, coronal, and sagittal views.

The MRI is especially useful in some areas where CT is not very
sensitive; these include the posterior fossa, the temporal bone, and
the skull base generally, where bone artifact limits the information
that CT is able to provide. MRI is also good for obtaining images of
the spinal canal, early white matter abnormalities such as low-grade
astrocytomas, small infarcts, multiple sclerosis, brain edema, spinal
intramedullary tumors, disc diseases, and syrinxes (Fig. 2.8). CT is
superior in assessing calcification and bone changes and in detecting
acute hemorrhages. CT is also less expensive and takes less time to
perform. Because of MRI's magnetic field, it is also not possible to
study patients with pacemakers or implanted foreign bodies contain-

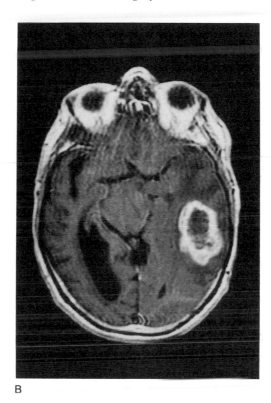

B

Figure 2.6. (continued)

ing ferrous material, nor those on life support systems with ferro-magnetic devices.

Objects that are whiter on MRI are said to have an increased signal, and those that are darker are said to have a decreased signal. Other important concepts in MRI are the terms T1- and T2-weighting and proton density. The physics involved can be complicated. Basically, proton density refers to the number of water molecules or of nuclear signals that are detected in the area of interest. The T1 time refers to the time it takes for return to original alignment of the particles that had been stimulated. Water and other liquids have long T1 times. The T1 time increases with increased field strength. T2 is a measure of the rate of loss of magnetization. Flow rate and direction also affect the signal. Most MRI studies include a T1-, a T2-,

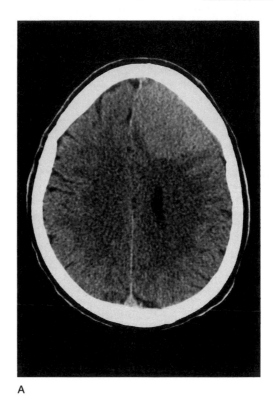

A

Figure 2.7. (A) CT and (B) MRI of a patient with a left frontal meningioma.

and a proton-weighted image. The T1 image is best used to show anatomical detail; the T2 image is better at showing contrast between tissue types (with some loss of detail); and the proton density combines high resolution with improved contrast. Table 2.3 summarizes T1 and T2 findings. MRI is more sensitive to cerebral edema, contusions, and white matter changes than CT. The age of blood clots can also be approximated from the MRI appearance of the hematoma. Table 2.4 summarizes the MRI appearance of intracranial hemorrhages by time after the initial hemorrhage.

In the subacute hemorrhage, deoxyhemoglobin changes to methemoglobin as the red blood cells lyse. There are hemosiderin-laden macrophages in the rim. In the chronic state, there is free methemoglobin and hemosiderin-laden macrophages in the surrounding

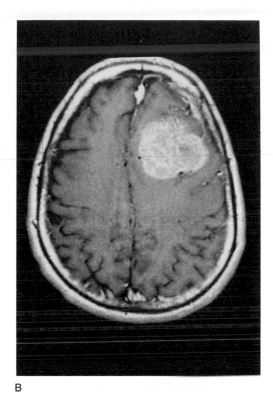

B

Figure 2.7. (continued)

tissue. These different stages of hemoglobin breakdown contribute to the MRI images described in Table 2.4.

Radioisotope Scanning

Since the advent of CT scanning, traditional technetium radioisotope scanning has been used infrequently. Its main application today is to show flow patterns that help diagnose brain death. It is also used to evaluate shunt function. Radioisotope is inserted into the CSF and the flow pattern is observed. Indium[111] cisternograms are also used to try to evaluate normal pressure hydrocephalus. An important new aspect of radioisotope scanning is single photon emis-

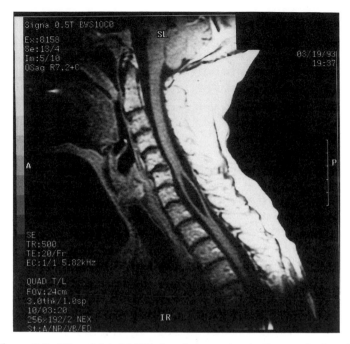

Figure 2.8. T1 weighted MRI showing a syrinx in the cervical cord.

Table 2.3. Signal Intensities on MRI

White on T1	Dark on T1
fat	CSF
white matter	flowing blood
contrast paramagnetic agents	edema or water
chronic blood	calcium
some tumors	gray matter
	some tumors

White on T2	Dark on T2
CSF	flowing blood
edema or water	calcium
contrast paramagnetic agents	white matter
MS plaques	acute blood
normal gray matter	fat
some tumors	some tumors
chronic blood	
inflammation	

Table 2.4. MRI Appearance of Blood

Time	T1 Image	T2 Image
Acute (less than 1 week)	Isointense	Hypointense center Isointense periphery Hyperintense edema of surrounding tissue
Subacute (7–30 days)	Isointense with some hypointensity in periphery	Hypointense with some isointensity in periphery and hyperintense edema of surrounding tissue
Chronic (over 30 days to 1 year)	Hyperintense with isointense surrounding tissue	Hyperintense with hypointense rim and isointense tissue

sion computed tomography (SPECT); its use is described in the next chapter.

Suggestions for Further Reading

Brant-Zawadsky M and Norman D. *Magnetic Resonance Imaging of the Central Nervous System.* New York: Raven Press, 1987.

Duvernoy H. *The Human Brain: Surface, Three-dimensional Sectional Anatomy and MRI.* Vienna: Springer-Verlag, 1991.

Heinz ER. Neuroradiology, Vol. 4. In Rosenberg RN, *The Clinical Neurosciences.* New York: Churchhill Livingston, 1984.

Osborn AG. *Introduction to Cerebral Angiography.* Hagerstown, Md.: Harper & Row, 1980.

Rubin JM and Chandler WF. *Ultrasound in Neurosurgery.* New York: Raven Press, 1989.

Shapiro R. *Myelography.* Chicago: Year Book, Fourth ed., 1984.

3

---

*Physiological Diagnosis
in Neurosurgery*

Introduction

Structural abnormalities in the nervous system can often be visualized radiologically, but increasing attention has been paid to imaging of nervous system function with other methods. This chapter describes several diagnostic methods that attempt to delineate nervous system function as well as structure. These include the electroencephalogram (EEG) and evoked responses, electromyograph (EMG) and nerve conduction studies, electronystagmograph (ENG), cerebral blood flow assessment, PET and SPECT scanning, and intracranial pressure monitoring.

The Electroencephalogram (EEG) and Evoked Responses

The electroencephalogram records electrical activity from the brain. Electrodes are pasted in different positions over the scalp and the changes in potential differences between them are recorded on a multichannel recorder as a function of time. The precise arrays of cells that generate the electrical activity are not known with certainty, but they probably represent impulses originating below the cerebral cortex. The brainstem and cerebellum, however, probably contribute nothing to the EEG. In a normal EEG pattern, four different kinds of electrical activity can be identified: alpha, 8–13 cycles per second (hertz) in the 20–60 microvolt range, especially characteristic of the occipital region in the rested but waking state; beta, 14–40 hertz, indicating arousal; theta in the 4 to 7 hertz range; and delta from 0.5 to 3 hertz. During sleep there are other normal complexes including sleep spindles.

Abnormal waves can be divided into two types: those indicating overactivity such as the irregular, violent pattern of a seizure; and slow waves, either delta or slower, which indicate decreased brain activity. Some medications characteristically suppress the EEG; the most common are barbiturates, but any tranquilizer can do this.

The EEG is most useful in assessing asymmetries of neurological activity, in identifying sites of abnormal electrical discharge, and in determining whether there is electrical activity at all (i.e., whether brain death has occurred). CT and MR scanning are superior to EEG in demonstrating a structural lesion; however, focal EEG asymmetries may be discovered in a patient thought to have diffuse neurological abnormalities, as in a patient suspected of having metabolic causes for coma who in fact has a chronic subdural hematoma or early infarct. Furthermore, EEG signs of seizure activity may be identified in patients with focal disorders, behavioral disturbances, or coma. The EEG is also used to monitor patients under anesthesia who are having carotid endarterectomy.

Computer techniques have modified the display of EEG activity; it can now be displayed as compressed power analysis or brain electrical activity mapping (BEAM). More importantly, the EEG response to a stimulus applied to one of the sense organs can be separated from remaining activity to give a summated response "evoked" by the stimulus. This response can provide a rough idea of the conduction in a particular anatomical pathway. Three evoked responses are commonly used: the visual evoked response (VER), usually to a pattern shift stimulus, which measures the time taken to conduct an impulse from retina to occipital lobe; the brainstem auditory evoked response (BAER) to a clicking noise, which tests the brainstem pathways from the cochlea to the temporal lobe; and the somatosensory evoked response (SSER), which tests the dorsal columns of the spinal cord and medial lemniscal pathways to the somatosensory cortex. The stimulus for the SSER is a repetitive tactile stimulus applied either to the peroneal nerve territory in the leg or to median nerve territory in the hand. The most useful measurement is the time taken for impulses to travel between certain points that can be readily identified. Prolongations are the chief abnormalities detectable, but amplitude may also be important; both can imply a disruption of normal anatomical pathways. Specific ranges of normal should be obtained in each electrophysiological unit doing these tests.

The Electromyogram and Nerve Conduction Studies

The electromyogram (EMG) and nerve conduction studies are methods of evaluating the resting and action potentials in individual muscles and nerves. The EMG relies on the fact that characteristic electrical patterns are associated with certain muscle abnormalities. Partial loss of nerve supply, for example, produces denervation potentials characterized by brief outbursts of low voltage activity. Structural muscle abnormalities may have specific discharge patterns, as in myotonic dystrophy. A knowledge of muscle supply and nerve pathways allows the delineation of regions of denervation in evaluating peripheral nerve disease.

The EMG has been most useful in diagnosing primary muscle diseases, including muscular dystrophies. In lumbar and cervical radiculopathy it may be useful if there is a question of establishing that there is denervation of one specific root or of distinguishing one root from another; however, denervation changes take several weeks to develop, so the EMG is not very useful in acute radiculopathy. Changes of denervation persist even after root decompression, making the tests less applicable in the diagnosis of persistent or recurrent pain.

Nerve conduction studies (NCS) evaluate the time taken for an impulse to travel from a stimulation point to particular sites along the nerve fiber path. Because of the variety of conduction velocities in a typical nerve, they may not be indicative of problems affecting specific fibers. They are most helpful in three situations: suspected compression along a peripheral nerve as occurs in ulnar, median, or peroneal compressive neuropathy; acute nerve injury in which a distinction between complete division and compression is important; and certain neuropathies where the myelin sheath is particularly affected. With both EMG and NCS it is helpful to discuss the clinical picture with the physician doing the test.

Cerebral Blood Flow

Cerebral blood flow techniques are still experimental. The most reliable types involve inhalation of radiolabeled xenon, sampling from arterial and venous blood, and calculation of xenon uptake in particular brain regions. These may show areas of hypoperfusion in stroke, and characteristic patterns have been suggested for a number of conditions, including acute hydrocephalus and Alzheimer's disease.

Doppler testing of arterial flow is a bedside test which may be useful in evaluating vasospasm in the ICU.

Intracranial Pressure Monitoring

Direct intracranial pressure (ICP) monitoring can be done by ventricular cannulation, insertion of a subarachnoid bolt, or insertion of an intraparenchymal fiberoptic monitor. The ventricular catheter system has the greatest accuracy but the risk of ventriculitis is higher. Intraparenchymal monitoring systems are accurate and have a lower infection rate.

There are three important forms of ICP waves. Normally there is a wave with fast upstroke and gradual decay, representing the arterial pulse with venous changes superimposed. This wave is superimposed on respiratory variation and represents normal ICP. Lundberg's "A" waves or plateau waves are prolonged elevations of ICP lasting over 5 minutes that achieve values twice the resting pressure; they are always abnormal and generally occur in a setting of increased ICP. Lundberg's "B" waves are elevations that are smaller and shorter than A waves. B waves do not have the same sinister significance as "A" waves.

Positron Emission Tomography Scanning

Like blood flow evaluation, positron emission tomography (PET) scanning is an experimental tool that combines physiological evaluation with anatomical display. A radiolabeled isotope, usually oxygen, is given intravenously and its metabolic distribution is charted by means of transaxial sections much like CT. With different isotopes, different patterns of function can be demonstrated. The place of PET scanning in neurosurgery is not yet certain. Equipment and isotopes are expensive, and the amount of information PET adds to more available imaging techniques is uncertain. The hope is that for cerebral ischemia it may show a deficit earlier than structural changes of the CT scan, thus allowing early treatment. For tumors PET scanning might also refine present diagnostic methods, correlating with stage of malignancy and also differentiating tumor from necrosis. For seizure disorders in children, there is some evidence that PET may show foci not recognized by electroencephalographic recording. At present, PET scanning is not useful in everyday practice.

Single Positron Emission Computed Tomography Scanning

Single positron emission computed tomography (SPECT) utilizes common isotopes found in nuclear medicine departments. Images are obtained in axial, coronal, and sagittal planes: three-dimensional images can also be reconstructed. Isotopes used include Technetium-99 HmPAO, thallium-201 chloride, and technetium-99 labeled red blood cells, but there are also a number of newer agents. After intravenous injection, Technetium-99 HmPAO is taken up by lipophilic cells such as brain cells in proportion to blood flow. Ischemic areas have a decreased uptake of this isotope, so it may prove useful in evaluating strokes. Thallium-201 chloride, a potassium analogue, is taken up by cells in proportion to cellular activity. This isotope is used to assess the integrity of the blood-brain barrier, which is disrupted by neoplasms. Tumors have an increased uptake of this agent, whereas regions of radiation necrosis have a low uptake of thallium. SPECT scanning with this agent is a promising tool in helping to distinguish between recurrence of tumor cells and necrosis. Another SPECT modality, Technetium-99 conjugated to red blood cells, is used to visualize vascular abnormalities such as arteriovenous malformations, venous angiomas, and cavernous angiomas.

Suggestions for Further Reading

Daly DD and Pedley TA. *Current Practice of Clinical Electroencephalography*. Second ed. New York: Raven Press, 1990.
Freedman AH, Drayer BP, and Jaszczak RJ. Single photon tomography. In Wilkins RH and Rengachary SS, *Neurosurgery*. New York: McGraw-Hill, 1985, pp. 265–267.

Ginsberg MD. Positron emission tomography. In Wilkins RH and Renga-
    chary SS, *Neurosurgery*. New York: McGraw-Hill, 1985, pp.
    255–264.
Johnson EW. *Electromyography*. Second ed. Baltimore: Williams & Wil-
    kins, 1988.
Kimura J. *Electrodiagnosis in Diseases of Nerve and Muscle: Principles
    and Practice*. Second ed. Philadelphia: FA Davis, 1989.

4

Differential Diagnosis of Common Neurosurgical Problems

This chapter presents several of the most frequent complaints or findings encountered in neurosurgery, emphasizing their differential diagnosis and neurosurgical implications.

Headache

The evaluation of headache requires careful history taking and examination, with attention to previous episodes, family history, exacerbating and relieving factors, distribution and radiation of pain, and accompanying symptoms and signs, such as papilledema. The neurosurgeon should recognize several characteristic types, keeping in mind that intracranial masses can mimic any of them.

Tension headache is the most common type of headache, affecting 80 percent or more of the population at some time. It is bilateral, dull, and poorly responsive to analgesics. Migraine has two forms, classic and common. *Classic migraine* affects young people, who usually have a family history, and presents with nausea, vomiting, irritability, a throbbing unilateral headache lasting 1–2 days, and contralateral visual disturbances such as field cuts and scintillations. It may be precipitated by bright light, certain foods, noise, or alcohol, and may be relieved by analgesics or sleep. *Common migraine* comprises 80 percent of migraines. It has a poorly defined prodrome of vague symptoms and presents as unilateral or bilateral headache, provoked by loud noise or bright light and relieved by sleep. Both kinds of migraine may be helped by prophylactic propranolol, or acutely treated with ergotamine at the onset. Dihydroergotamine mesylate (DHE), an ergot derivative, is also useful in the acute management of these headaches. *"Cluster"* headaches usually occur in men and are characterized by relatively brief unilateral retroorbital pain at night associated with eye tearing and nasal congestion. They occur repeatedly for many days; ergotamine 2 mg at bedtime may prevent them. These specific headache syndromes may not need further workup if diagnosed properly.

Other headache syndromes must be recognized because of their potentially serious import. Headache of sudden onset with neck stiffness in a patient without previous headaches should be considered symptomatic of subarachnoid hemorrhage or meningitis until proven otherwise. The headache need not be severe but should be investigated with CT followed by lumbar puncture if the CT does not show a mass or intracranial bleed.

Headache that is worse in the morning, or generalized and accompanied by vomiting and nausea that does not fit a migraine pattern, is a common symptom of increased intracranial pressure. It requires careful neurological examination and ideally a CT scan with contrast enhancement.

Facial pain occurring on one side of the face with a lancinating quality often precipitated by light touch to the face is likely to be trigeminal neuralgia. Occipital neuralgia may have the same quality but be distributed in the posterior scalp unilaterally.

Weakness

Muscular weakness can signify neurological disturbance anywhere from muscle to cerebral cortex. In making the diagnosis, it is helpful to begin by deciding whether the disorder affects muscle itself, the neuromuscular junction, the anterior horn cell and its axons, or the descending tracts that influence the anterior horn cell's activity. A history of cramping, paresthesia, or bladder disorder; findings of muscle wasting, changes in muscle tone, sensory loss, or fasciculations; patterns of weakness; and tests of serum enzymes, EMG and muscle biopsy may help separate these possibilities.

Primary muscle disorders are generally characterized by diffuse proximal weakness; atrophy; loss of reflexes; diminished tone; elevation of serum enzymes including creatinine, phosphatase, SGOT, and SGPT; specific findings on EMG; and on biopsy a random pattern of degeneration or regeneration, as well as characteristic histochemical staining abnormalities in specific disorders. Examples of such muscle disorders are the muscular dystrophies, periodic paralyses, glycogen or carbohydrate storage diseases, and congenital or drug-induced myopathies.

Disorders of the neuromuscular junction, such as myasthenia gravis, are characterized by fluctuating weakness without atrophy. Reflexes are preserved. There are distinctive amplitude changes (a "fatigue" pattern) on repetitive stimulation in nerve conduction studies.

Disorders of the anterior horn cell can be divided into those affecting the nerve cell body itself and those affecting the axon in the peripheral nerve. These are both components of the lower motor neuron, whose loss is characterized by flaccid weakness, decreased tone, muscle wasting, and fasciculations. Disorders affecting anterior horn cell bodies are spinal disorders with a pattern of weakness, muscle wasting, hyporeflexia, and fasciculations that follow innervation segments (e.g. C7, T2, etc.). The EMG and muscle biopsy will show so called "neuropathic" changes consisting of fibrillations at rest, diminished interference pattern on EMG, and a "grouped fiber" pattern of atrophy on biopsy. Examples of anterior horn cell body disorders are poliomyelitis and Werdnig-Hoffman sclerosis. Amyotrophic lateral sclerosis, which affects upper as well as lower motor neurons, may produce the same symptoms as well as hyperreflexia. Disorders affecting the axon of the anterior horn cell are peripheral nerve diseases characterized by paresthesias and sensory loss, as well as weakness, atrophy and hyporeflexia of muscles supplied by specific nerves, slowed nerve conduction velocity, and the same neuropathic changes that are seen in diseases affecting the cell body. CSF protein may be elevated.

"Upper motor neuron weakness" results from abnormalities above the anterior horn cell in the spinal cord, brain stem, or cortical motor tracts. It is characterized by increased limb tone with hyperactive reflexes and Babinski's sign. There is no fasciculation and the weakness always occurs in large muscle groups rather than in a single muscle or nerve supply. Nerve conduction studies and EMG are normal.

Associated findings may indicate where the lesion is. With spinal cord lesions the weakness is usually bilateral with a corresponding sensory level. With brain stem lesions there is usually an abnormality of the cranial nerves. In cortical disorders the weakness is unilateral, often affects an entire limb, and is not consistently accompanied by loss of pinprick sensation, light touch, or joint position sense.

Causes of *rapidly progressive flaccid weakness* with no sensory or bladder loss include Guillain-Barre syndrome, early spinal cord compression, tick paralysis, acute viral or idiopathic polymyositis, malignant hyperpyrexia (neuroleptic malignant syndrome), "alcoholic" polymyopathy, acute paroxysmal hemoglobinuria, and fulminant myasthenia gravis. Episodic muscle weakness occurs in hypo- and hyperkalemic periodic paralyses, characterized by potassium shifts, and in myasthenia gravis, including Eaton Lambert syndrome.

Chronic diffuse muscle wasting can be caused by three categories of disease: muscle, spinal root, and peripheral nerve. The progressive muscular dystrophies, chronic polymyositis, and chronic myopathies are examples of the first category. Infantile muscle atrophy (Werdnig-Hoffman disease), amyotrophic lateral sclerosis, and a variety of other progressive muscle atrophies are in the second group. In the third group (peripheral nerve disease) it is important to distinguish chronic neural atrophies such as Charcot-Marie-Tooth disease, chronic nutritional polyneuropathy, hypertrophic polyneuritis, and leprosy. Some of these diseases will also need to be distinguished from spinal cord tumors.

Weakness of one arm without atrophy is usually of cortical origin, although an early stage of a spinal disorder is possible. With atrophy, its occurrence in an infant suggests brachial plexus disease. Weakness of one leg is usually the result of intervertebral disc disease, trauma, tumor, or multiple sclerosis.

Spastic hemiplegia, weakness of both arm and leg on one side, is common. It can result from upper motor neuron lesions in the cortex, brain stem, or rarely spinal cord. Seizures, aphasia or field defects are associated with cortical lesions. Cranial palsies accompany brain stem lesions, and spinal cord lesions usually produce disorders on both sides of the body.

Paraplegia usually arises from spinal cord disease. Paraplegia developing over a few minutes virtually always means spinal cord trauma, infarct, or hemorrhage. Paraplegia developing over hours may have one of several causes: epidural abscess, hematoma, or tumor are the most significant neurosurgically. Their separation from multiple sclerosis, postinfectious myelitis, neurosyphilis myelitis, poliomyelitis, and Guillain-Barre syndrome will require myelography or MRI in most cases, and this must be done expeditiously. In infants, paraparesis is often seen as delay in starting to walk. It can result from birth trauma to the spinal cord or head, muscle disease, neuron disorders, or congenital lesions of brain or spinal cord. Chronic progressive paraplegia has many causes. In children, spinal cord tumors such as lymphoma and ependymoma, and congenital spine anomalies including tethered cord, must be considered. Other causes to be considered include Friedreich's ataxia, progressive muscular dystrophy, and chronic polyneuropathy. In adults, neurosurgically important causes of chronic progressive paraplegia include spinal cord or vertebral column tumors, cervical disc or osteophyte, chronic epidural infection, and syringomyelia. These must be distinguished from multiple sclerosis, subacute combined degeneration, syphilis, amyotrophic lateral sclerosis, polyneuritis, and polymyositis.

Sensory Loss

Loss of sensation can follow the distribution of a peripheral nerve, a spinal root (dermatome), an entire spinal cord section (segment), or the cortex (a limb). Causes of sensory loss in a segmental or dermatomal distribution can conveniently be grouped by age. In children and young adults a congenital anomaly of the spine, an intervertebral disc rupture, or a tumor (especially a neurofibroma) are most likely. In adults, the cause depends somewhat on the region affected. In the lumbar and sacral roots, dermatomal pain or loss of sensation is most likely caused by disc disease; tumor and diabetic neuropathy are other possibilities. In the neck, spondylitic change is most common. Tumor, AVM and syrinx are also possible causes. Thoracic outlet syndromes and brachial plexopathies are hard to separate from these conditions at times. Segmental pain in the thorax usually arises from an extramedullary tumor or disc. An arteriovenous malformation, herpes zoster, B12 deficiency, and multiple sclerosis must also be considered.

Loss of sensation in a single limb has quite a different set of possible causes. If more than one root is involved, disease of the plexus supplying the limb must be considered; this may be a plexopathy, intrinsic or extrinsic tumor, or other mass. Nerve entrapment or nerve tumor can also produce analgesia or anesthesia in one limb. Sensory loss in one modality but not another ("dissociated" loss) implies a spinal cord or brain stem lesion, usually a syrinx. Symmetrical, distal primary sensory loss in the limb usually implies a peripheral neuropathy. This "glove and stocking" anesthesia may be caused by any neuropathy.

Back and Leg Pain

Back pain may emanate from bony, ligamentous, muscular, disc, or neural elements. In infants and young children, back pain may represent inflammatory disorders such as discitis or abscess, or even early meningitis; tumor; or, less commonly, disc herniation. In those aged from 10–20, it suggests tumor. In adults aged 20–40, the most common variety is postural pain, with disc herniation second and primary bony neoplasm third. In older adults the most common cause is spondylosis; other causes include metabolic bone disease, metastatic tumor, epidural or subdural abscess, herniated disc, intraspinal hematoma, and acute myelitis.

Pain involving both the back and the leg has a different set of causes than back pain alone. These include disorders of nerve roots, lumbosacral plexus, sciatic nerve, and other pelvic structures (see Table 4.1). Root compression can be caused by disc, bone, abscess, hematoma, or tumor. Pain arising from structural spinal column defects is usually unmodified by activity; in evaluating such pain, it is very important to obtain a myelogram or MRI that includes the conus. This will help to exclude a mass compressing a root outside the canal. Paresthesia rather than pain suggests root compression outside the spinal canal.

Pelvic lesions can be assessed by careful rectal and pelvic examinations and CT of the pelvis. Vascular lesions are discernable by loss of pedal pulses, history of claudication, and noninvasive vascular testing. Both may mimic disc disease.

Neck, Shoulder, and Arm Pain

The differential diagnosis of pain in the neck, shoulder and arm must include diseases of the spine, the brachial plexus, and the shoulder joint itself. Pain arising from the spinal column or spinal cord is felt in the neck and the back of the head; it is exacerbated by head move-

Table 4.1. Causes of Radicular Back Pain

A. Lumbar Root Compression in the Spinal Canal
   1. Extradural root compression
      a. disc rupture
      b. osteophyte
      c. ligamentous or fibrotic constriction
      d. vertebral abscess or tumor
      e. extradural hematoma
   2. Nerve root tumor or cyst
   3. Arteriovenous malformation of conus or root
B. Lumbosacral Plexus Lesion
   1. Pelvic infection
   2. Pelvic neoplasm
   3. Sacroiliac joint lesion, inflammation, or injury
   4. Endometriosis
   5. Trauma to plexus
C. Sciatic Nerve Lesion
   1. Contusion, including hematoma or direct injury
   2. Neoplasm
   3. Inflammation
      a. toxic
      b. infective
      c. viral
      d. metabolic
D. Referred Pain
   1. From disc degeneration
   2. From sacroiliac joint
   3. From arthritis of the hip joint
   4. From Baker's cyst of the popliteal fossa
   5. From the femur
E. Vascular Problems
   1. Tibial compartmental syndrome
   2. Peripheral vascular disease
F. Thalamic or Other "Central" Pain

ment and accompanied by cervical muscle spasm and tenderness. It may be associated with paresthesias, sensory loss, weakness, or deep tendon reflex change. Although disc disease or spondylosis are most common, the possibility of syringomyelia, amyotrophic lateral sclerosis, or cervical tumor must also be kept in mind and may only be excluded by myelography or MRI.

    Pain originating in the brachial plexus is felt in the shoulder and supraclavicular regions. A cervical rib or fibrous band may compress the plexus as part of the thoracic outlet syndrome, a difficult and sometimes overused diagnosis. A tumor of the apex of the lung

(Pancoast tumor) must be considered as well when assessing the cause of arm pain.

Pain of shoulder origin is often worse at night and is associated with tenderness; it is worse on shoulder movement. Tendonitis or bursitis is the most common problem; there are no sensory, motor, or reflex changes. Carpal tunnel or ulnar entrapment may cause shoulder and arm pains; reflex sympathetic dystrophy, rheumatoid arthritis, osteoarthritis, neuritis, and neuralgia may also cause arm pain.

Gait Disturbances

Gait disturbances can be roughly classified by age. In infants, difficulty starting to walk is rarely attributable to neurosurgical causes, but the rare cases are from increasing intracranial pressure, hydrocephalus, chronic subdural hematoma, tumor, or degenerative disease. In children, gait trouble may be caused by Friedreich's ataxia, spinocerebellar degeneration, hydrocephalus, chronic subdural hematoma, brain or spinal cord tumor, or defect of spinal formation. In young adults, multiple sclerosis and spinal tumor are the most common causes. In older patients, amyotrophic lateral sclerosis, spondylosis, and high spinal tumor are important causes. In patients over age 50, Parkinson's disease, diffuse encephalopathy, and normal pressure hydrocephalus are also possible causes.

Drowsiness, Stupor, and Coma

These terms describe changes in the level of consciousness that are important in neurosurgical evaluation. In recording these changes, it is more important to describe precise responses to stimuli than to speak of "obtundation" or "stupor." The Glasgow coma scale (p. 64) is one easily reproduced method of assessing overall responsiveness.

Drowsiness can be caused by medications, recreational drugs, metabolic or systemic disorders, mass lesions, or inflammations of brain and meninges. Among the medications that may reduce alertness are anticonvulsants, antihistamines, antihypertensives, analgesics, antidepressants, anxiolytics, and soporifics. Some metabolic causes of impaired mental status include hypoxia, hypo- or hyperthermia, hypoglycemia, hormonal deficits, ion imbalances, and infection. Postoperative obtundation is often especially difficult to assess: in a previously brain injured or elderly patient, anesthetic effects may last for a prolonged period. Their effect is usually symmetrical so that they can be differentiated from mass lesions.

Inflammatory disorders of the brain that may alter the state of consciousness include subarachnoid hemorrhage, meningitis, and encephalitis. In these conditions, neck stiffness plus an abnormal cerebrospinal fluid cell count are the distinguishing features.

Mass lesions causing drowsiness are especially important for the neurosurgeon. The frontal, cerebellar, and parietal regions are treacherous because lesions in these areas may produce only drowsiness without other signs. This is also true for intraventricular tumors, which may cause hydrocephalus and drowsiness without other signs. Intracerebral hemorrhage, infarction, epidural or subdural hematoma, brain tumor, brain abscess, and subdural empyema are among the causes of drowsiness that are relevant to neurosurgeons. They usually, but not always, produce asymmetrical motor or sensory findings.

There are several less common causes of drowsiness. Infarcts of the smaller perforating branches of the circle of Willis may do so without marked mass effect, as may cerebral contusions and seizures.

Strokes and TIAs

The sudden onset of a cerebrovascular deficit that is called stroke may represent one of several events in the nervous system. About one-third of strokes are brain infarcts associated with atherosclerosis in the carotid artery. Twenty percent of strokes result from cardiac or other emboli, 20 percent from abnormalities in small intraparenchymal atherosclerotic vessels associated with hypertension and lacunar infarct, 10 percent from intracerebral hemorrhage, and 10 percent from ruptured aneurysms. Examination of the cardiac rhythm and pulses of vessels in the neck, auscultation of the heart and great vessels, measurement of arterial blood pressure, and assessment of peripheral vasculature are important in distinguishing these different causes of stroke. A stroke whose symptoms increase for 6 hours or more is especially suggestive of intracranial hematoma or tumor and requires urgent neurosurgical evaluation.

Transient ischemic attacks (TIAs) are episodes of temporary focal cerebral dysfunction lasting less than 24 hours. They can be caused by either carotid or vertebrobasilar ischemia. Aphasia, hemiparesis, monocular blindness (amaurosis fugax) and hemisensory disturbance are characteristic of carotid territory ischemia. Visual field disturbances, vertigo, and drop attacks are characteristic of vertebrobasilar ischemia. Steadily progressive deficit over hours suggests an intracranial hematoma; sudden headache and deficit with stiff neck suggests subarachnoid hemorrhage. Brain tumors and subdural hematomas can produce symptoms resembling those of an infarct, as can seizure disorders.

In the diagnosis of stroke, MRI is the most sensitive early detector for parenchymal ischemic stroke but CT is more sensitive for hemorrhage. CT can exclude remediable hemorrhagic causes and therefore may be the best tool. Depending on the CT results and the clinical situation, lumbar puncture and arteriography may be necessary.

Dizziness

Dizziness, like headache, is a common and difficult-to-diagnose complaint. The most important initial step in its evaluation is to try to determine whether true vertigo is part of the symptoms. Vertigo implies the illusory sensation of spinning either of the patient himself or of his surroundings. It can be of peripheral origin (from the peripheral portion of the vestibular nerve) or of central origin (from the vestibular nucleus). Ninety percent of vertigo is peripheral, but the central causes are more serious and therefore must be looked for carefully. With a peripheral lesion, significant vertigo is accompanied by nystagmus. It generally lasts fewer than 3 weeks and has associated auditory phenomena.

Vertigo of peripheral origin may be caused by cerebellopontine angle tumors; vertebrobasilar insufficiency; Meniere's disease (characterized by an aura of tinnitus, sensorineural hearing loss, and head pressure on the affected side with distortion of sound followed by sudden, severe, whirling vertigo); vestibular neuronitis (characterized by absent caloric response in the affected ear, absence of other symptoms, and short duration of 1 to 3 weeks); benign paroxysmal positional vertigo (characterized by vertigo only with certain head positions, and by gross vertigo and nystagmus that can be elicited by placing the head in the position responsible); labyrinthitis either of serous type or from acute bacterial infection; toxic labyrinthine injury from streptomycin, vancomycin, ethacrynic acid, gentamycin, kanamycin, neomycin, or nitrogen mustard; and vertigo from neck injury or spasm. In the last case, there is limited cervical motion and palpable spasm of the cervical musculature.

With central lesions nystagmus often is greater than vertigo and is associated with other signs of brain stem dysfunction. Important central causes of vertigo include epilepsy, in which the vertigo occurs as part of the aura in 16 percent of cases; multiple sclerosis; posterior fossa metastasis; and thrombosis of a posterior fossa artery.

Dizziness that lacks vertigo's true feeling of rotation or impulsion is difficult to evaluate. The sensation is usually described as swaying, light-headedness, or feeling "about to pass out." It may be a manifestation of anxiety or depression but its general causes have not been satisfactorily described.

Suggestions for Further Reading

Adams RD and Victor M. *Principles of Neurology,* Fourth ed. New York: McGraw-Hill, 1989.

DeJong RN. *The Neurologic Examination.* Fourth ed. Hagerston, Md.: Harper & Row, 1979.

Mayo Clinic Staff. *Clinical Examinations in Neurology.* Fifth ed. Philadelphia: W.B. Saunders, 1981.

Rowland LP. *Merritt's Textbook of Neurology.* Eighth ed. Philadelphia: Lea & Febiger, 1989, pp. 32–35.

II

Neurosurgical Management

This section reviews the general management of patients with neurosurgical disorders. Emergency situations that are often encountered by neurosurgeons are discussed in Chapter 5. Drugs frequently used in neurosurgery are reviewed in Chapter 6. A discussion of common neurosurgical procedures, an outline of management protocols, and a brief account of complications in neurosurgery are then presented in Chapters 7, 8, and 9.

5

Neurosurgical Emergencies

This chapter discusses pathological processes encountered in neurosurgery that require prompt recognition and treatment on the part of the neurosurgeon. Topics presented include head trauma, herniation syndromes, spinal cord injury, paraplegia or quadriplegia, ataxia, coma, status epilepticus, meningitis, and cardiac arrest.

Acute Head Trauma

Head trauma may have a variety of sequelae from transient loss of consciousness to irreversible coma. Acute head injuries are classified as mild, moderate, or severe. In *mild* head injury, the patient has a history of trauma but feels well except for such symptoms as headache or dizziness. In *moderate* head injury, the patient may have manifestations of increased intracranial pressure such as nausea and vomiting but can obey commands. In *severe* head injury, the patient cannot obey commands. Patients with severe head injury and those with progressive neurological dysfunction are neurosurgical emergencies. The Glasgow Coma Scale (GCS) (see Table 5.1) is a useful schema for rating the severity of injury. It provides a basis both for initial evaluation and for sequential follow-up by others. The essential elements include the best motor response, the best verbal response, and the stimulus required for eye opening. The total score is obtained by adding the scores for each section (E + M + V).

Table 5.1. The Glasgow Coma Scale

Eye opening (E)	
opens eyes spontaneously	4
opens eyes to voice	3
opens eyes to pain	2
no eye opening	1
Best motor response (in best limb) (M)	
obeys commands	6
localizes to pain	5
withdraws to pain	4
abnormal flexion	3
abnormal extension	2
no movement	1
Best verbal response (V)	
appropriate and oriented	5
confused conversation	4
inappropriate words	3
incomprehensible sounds	2
no sounds	1

(T) is used if the patient has a tracheostomy.

Mild Head Injury

Mild head injuries include scalp trauma and concussion. A concussion is a transient loss of consciousness or neurological function. Patients in this category usually have a GCS of 13–15. About one in ten patients with a GCS of 13–15 will have an abnormal CT scan, about 3 percent requiring surgery. More importantly, about four in ten patients with a GCS of less than 13 will have an abnormal CT scan, about 13 percent of whom will require surgery.

A CT scan is recommended for patients who are symptomatic after their head injury or who lose conciousness for more than 5 minutes; history or physical exam alone may not be adequate to assess the risk of worsening. A GCS of 14 to 15 and a normal CT predicts a good outcome, and these patients can be discharged to home observation with an appropriate set of instructions about what to watch for. In patients over 60 or under 5 years of age, evidence of alcohol ingestion, other injuries, persistent nausea and vomiting, the absence of reliable family members or friends to observe the patient at home, an abnormal CT scan, or a GCS of 13 or less should usually indicate the need for hospitalization.

If a CT scanner is not available, documented loss of consciousness for over 5 minutes usually mandates overnight observation. Shorter periods of unconsciousness are best approached by assessing the patient's condition, including symptoms of headache, dizziness, vomiting, ataxia, or evidence of skull fracture. If the patient is neurologically intact and those around him seem reliable, discharge with written instructions describing changes to watch for may be appropriate. Such a sheet should usually be given when any patient with a head injury is discharged from the emergency room. Taking an apparent mild head injury seriously will not only help make the initial exclusion of major lesions but also will help if there are delayed symptoms.

Moderate Head Injury

Patients in this category have a GCS of 9–12. A CT scan is mandatory along with hourly observation in an intensive care unit. Subsequent management depends on the development of further symptoms and signs.

Severe Head Injury

Patients in this category have a GCS of 8 or less, and should have an immediate CT scan. Management is directed at making an accurate diagnosis of intracranial problems that may need urgent decompressive surgery and avoiding further brain injury from hypoxia, hypotension, and cerebral edema.

Initial Evaluation

Management in the emergency room begins with the ABC's: evaluating and maintaining *a*irway, *b*reathing, and *c*irculation. This is immediately followed by a thorough general examination to assess potentially life-threatening injuries, a neurological examination, and definitive radiological studies including cervical spine evaluation. All patients should be transported on a backboard with cervical spine immobilization using sandbags or a Philadelphia collar.

AIRWAY.   In the prone, unconscious, or semiconscious patient, airway obstruction is commonly caused by the epiglottis and flaccid tongue falling posteriorly in the pharynx. Chin lift or jaw thrust with minimal cervical extension will open the airway safely even with an unstable cervical spine. In addition, the mouth should be quickly cleared of debris, vomit suctioned and any obstructing dentures removed. An oropharyngeal airway can then be placed.

BREATHING.   Standard cardiopulmonary resuscitation may have been done in the field by emergency medical technicians but should be reviewed on the patient's arrival in the emergency room. Resuscitation with mask and bag followed by careful intubation may be necessary. A good general rule is to intubate anyone who is obtunded enough to tolerate the endotracheal tube, preferably using nasotracheal intubation. A lateral cervical spine film should be obtained first to exclude a cervical fracture. If there is a cervical fracture, extensive facial injury, or obstacle to rapid intubation, a tracheostomy or cricothyrotomy may be necessary. Simultaneously, large-bore IVs are placed and arterial blood gases should be taken; the ventilator should be set to deliver an oxygen concentration to achieve a PaO_2 greater than 80 torr and a $PaCO_2$ of 30–35 torr. With signs of herniation, the patient is hyperventilated to achieve a $PaCO_2$ of 25–30 torr.

CIRCULATION.   If there is no pulse, standard external chest compression is begun followed immediately by the appropriate drugs or transthoracic electrical stimulation as outlined by the American Heart Association.

BLEEDING.   In adults, hypotension should not be considered a result of head injury until a thorough search for another source has been conducted. Thigh and abdomen are two regions to check. Hypotension accompanied by bradycardia and flaccid extremities may be an indication of concomitant spinal cord injury and spinal shock. In children, on the other hand, significant blood loss can occur from scalp lacerations or bleeding into the subdural space, and hypotension may result from this.
    Volume resuscitation is best accomplished with blood products when there is a hematocrit below 28. While cross-match is proceeding, fluids that minimize free water administration (e.g. 5% dextrose/normal saline, 5% dextrose/0.45% normal saline) should be used to minimize brain swelling exacerbated by hypotonic fluids.

CERVICAL SPINE INJURY. Cervical spine injury should always be assumed in the severely head-injured patient. Immobilization with a collar, sandbags, or backboard is imperative until adequate X-rays (usually portable lateral cervical spine) have excluded spine injury from occiput through C7. Often C_1 to C_2 and C_7 are poorly visualized and cannot be read as normal. In these cases the collar/immobilization should stay in place. During CT scanning for head injury, the C1 and C7 levels can also be scanned to exclude fracture.

General Examination

The general physical examination should establish the extent of chest, abdominal, and long bone injuries, identify any sites of hemorrhage, and lead to further consultation when indicated. Careful examination of the scalp and face, looking for abrasions, foreign bodies, lacerations, punctures, and drainage of spinal fluid from nose or ear should be followed by more formal neurological testing to establish the level of consciousness and asymmetry of function.

Neurological History

Every attempt should be made to establish the initial mechanism and severity of injury, evidence of prolonged anoxia or hypotension, neurological status at the scene and any subsequent change, and seizure activity or drug or alcohol use. This information can provide the neurosurgeon with important clues to the patient's condition.

Neurological Examination

In the formal neurological evaluation, the most important features are: 1) the level of consciousness, 2) lateralization of motor or cranial nerve findings, suggesting a focal intracranial mass, 3) "brainstem" findings, suggesting primary or secondary brainstem injury, and 4) a change in the neurological picture over time. Neurological testing should include the Glasgow Coma Scale along with examination of asymmetry of motor response, deep tendon reflexes, extraocular movements, pupil size and reactivity, corneal response, gag, and respiratory pattern.

Assessing the *level of consciousness* includes the following: Does the patient follow commands? Speak when spoken to or when pinched? Brush the examiner away in response to a painful stimulus? Move to any stimulus?

Motor responses may give an important clue to asymmetry of function and to the level of injury. Diminished movement with increased deep tendon reflexes on one side suggests a focal brain injury. Rapidly developing decerebrate posturing, with internal rotation and extension of a limb, suggests an intracranial hematoma or other mass on the side of the brain opposite the posturing limb.

Eye opening, eye movement, and pupillary response can provide information on the level of consciousness as well as brain stem function. Eye movements normally fix upon and follow the examiner, suggesting both intact brainstem and cortex. Spontaneous conjugate roving eye movements imply intact brainstem function but cortical dysfunction. A lack of any spontaneous eye movements should be further evaluated by turning the head from side to side or irrigating the ear with 20 cc of ice water, which should cause conjugate eye deviation toward the side of stimulation. If there is no eye movement in response to this maneuver, severe brain stem injury or drug intoxication is likely. Pupils should be equal and reactive to light. Causes of an unreactive pupil include third nerve palsy, blindness, and an artificial eye. Unilateral pupillary dilatation in the comatose head-injured patient suggests third nerve or midbrain compression secondary to brain shifts caused by a mass lesion. Pupillary dilatation is ipsilateral to the mass approximately 90 percent of the time in the acute setting. Bilaterally dilated pupils indicate extensive primary or secondary midbrain injury. Very small pupils suggest pontine hemorrhage.

Lack of corneal or gag response suggests brainstem dysfunction. A common abnormal respiratory pattern is Cheyne-Stokes respiration, with waxing and waning and intermittent pauses; this suggests bilateral cerebral hemisphere injury. Anther characteristic pattern is hyperventilation, seen with pontine injury.

The trend of the neurologic state over time is extremely important, and serial examination should be performed and documented regularly. Neurological deterioration can signal an increase in the size of a hematoma or impending herniation.

Radiological Studies

In the severely head-injured patient, films in the emergency room should include a lateral cervical spine film that visualizes C_1 to T_1. It may be necessary to pull down the shoulders of husky patients or get "swimmer's views" to eliminate soft tissue obscuration of the lower cervical vertebrae.

A plain CT scan of the head is the radiographic procedure of choice in severe head injury. It rapidly and accurately identifies traumatic hemorrhage and provides information on the location and nature of intracranial masses. The extent of skull fractures and bony sinus involvement is estimated as well. Occasionally frontal-orbital and facial injuries are better seen with coronal views. Cervical spine "cuts" through C_7 may be done if it is not well visualized on the cervical spine film.

If a CT scan is unavailable, cerebral arteriography is a far less satisfactory second choice; it can show the nature and degree of shift from an intracranial mass but not whether the mass is due to contusion, swelling, or blood clot. If no CT scan is available within one hour, consideration should be given to rapid transfer to a facility with a CT immediately available. MRI is not as helpful as CT in acute head injury.

Lumbar puncture should *not* be performed in patients with severe head injury. The pressure gradient caused by removal of fluid from the lumbar subarachnoid space can lead to cerebral herniation and death in the presence of a mass lesion. Moreover, no useful information is provided by lumbar puncture.

Initial Resuscitation

One or two large-bore (16 gauge) intravenous catheters should be inserted expeditiously and blood should be drawn for prothrombin time, partial thromboplastin time, platelet count, electrolytes, sugar, blood urea nitrogen, and typing and cross-matching with a request for four units of packed cells. One tube is held for alcohol, toxic screen, or other testing. Lactated Ringer's or other isotonic intravenous (IV) fluid is administered at maintenance rate when there are no signs of herniation or hypotension. A Foley catheter is inserted into the bladder and arterial blood gases are drawn.

Correction of hypotension with volume replacement should be the first concern. If there is no hypotension, IV fluids such as normal saline or lactated Ringer's should be given sparingly. If there is focal injury, many surgeons give one gram of IV phenytoin mixed in normal saline as seizure prophylaxis upon the adult patient's arrival. The phenytoin must be given no faster than 50 mg/min. Dexamethasone as a means of reducing acute cerebral edema has little proven efficacy but is used in some centers.

If there is asymmetric movement or posturing (implying a mass lesion), one gram per kilogram body weight of mannitol solution should be given by IV push as fast as possible and a CT scan should be done immediately while a neurosurgeon is called. If there is a definite herniation syndrome (see below), immediate surgery may be necessary. It is important to know what arrangement the hospital has for this contingency before it occurs, as minutes may make the difference between good quality survival and persistent vegetative existence in these patients.

If the CT scan shows a mass with shift over 5–10 mm, surgery will probably be needed. If there is just diffuse swelling, intracranial pressure should be monitored in an intensive care unit (ICU).

Herniation Syndromes

Herniation syndromes suggest compression of the brainstem or other important structures against the fixed structures of the cranium (falx, tentorium) by a mass on one side of the brain. There are three types: lateral tentorial herniation, central tentorial herniation, and foramen magnum herniation. Each must be recognized and treated promptly.

Lateral Tentorial Herniation

The hallmark of lateral uncal tentorial herniation (compression of the brain stem by the uncus of the temporal lobe) is dilation of the ipsilateral pupil. In addition, there is usually increasing drowsiness or agitation, weakness followed by decorticate or decerebrate posturing of arm and leg on the side opposite the dilating pupil, hyperventilation, complete third nerve palsy, and incontinence. Pathophysiologically, this sequence represents third nerve and brainstem compression by the ipsilateral medial temporal lobe extending across the tentorial notch. Parasympathetic pupil fibers located circumferentially in the third nerve are lost early, producing a unilateral poorly responsive and dilating pupil. Posturing or weakness of limbs, usually contralateral to the pupillary enlargement, follows because of pyramidal tract compression in the brainstem on the side of an expanding lesion above the crossing of fibers in the pyramidal decussation.

The emergency management of this herniation syndrome is immediate intubation, hyperventilation, and intravenous mannitol

(1–2 g/kg) and Furosemide (.5 mg/kg) to shrink the surrounding brain. One or two transaxial sections of a CT scan may be made on the way to the operating room if they can be obtained quickly.

Central Herniation and Acute Hydrocephalus

The syndrome of central tentorial herniation is less obvious than the unilateral syndrome but is just as fatal. Here the entire brainstem is pushed down symmetrically; the third nerve may not be compressed. The pupils therefore may remain small and reactive while stupor becomes coma and motor responses deteriorate from hemiparesis to bilateral decerebrate rigidity. This syndrome presents as drowsiness without focal signs. As it progresses, there may be sighing or Cheyne-Stokes respiration, small reactive pupils, and decorticate posturing (arm flexion and leg extension) followed by bilateral decerebrate posturing. The treacherous feature is that there is rarely the dilated pupil of the unilateral syndrome. Untreated, central herniation progresses to foramen magnum herniation with medullary compromise, respiratory arrest, and death.

Although this syndrome can be caused by any bilateral central mass, the major cause is acute hydrocephalus supratentorially. If there is a history of hydrocephalus and clinical findings suggest central herniation, emergent ventriculostomy (or a shunt tap when applicable) should be considered even before diagnostic studies.

Foramen Magnum Herniation

Foramen magnum herniation is signaled by drowsiness, respiratory arrest, and death. It may occur as the last step in a central herniation syndrome, or it may occur alone with a posterior fossa mass. Usually there are signs of increased pressure in the posterior fossa: headache, neck stiffness, vomiting, and gait difficulty. These early signs must be recognized immediately because of the increased likelihood of fatality: CT scanning should be carried out urgently with special attention to the posterior fossa. This is one acute syndrome in whch MRI may demonstrate a lesion not well seen on CT because of bony artifact. Mannitol may temporize here but there is even less time than with tentorial termination as irreversible medullary injury is a likely sequel. The mass effect, whatever its nature, must be removed.

Acute Spinal Cord Injury

Initial Evaluation and Management

Spinal cord injury should be assumed in any patient with severe head injury until adequate radiological examination rules it out. In the victim of any trauma, vertebral column pain or tenderness, arm or leg tingling or weakness, neck deformity, or a history of these symptoms is presumptive evidence of spinal cord injury until excluded.

The initial care of spinal injury, like that of any other severe injury, involves assessment of immediate life-threatening problems: the ABC's—airway, breathing and circulation. Subsequent care is directed at anatomical alignment of the spine. Unlike head injuries, acute cervical spine injuries have different indications for immediate surgery because the damage appears to be irreversible within seconds of its occurrence.

Management and evaluation proceed together. The goals of management are to assure stable anatomical alignment, prevent further spinal cord injury, and support the patient physiologically. At the accident scene it is extremely important to determine whether spinal injury has occurred by assessing neck pain, postural deformity, spinal tenderness, and subjective or objective neurological changes in the trunk or extremities. The emergency medical technician needs to document response to painful stimulus and movement in all extremities. Patients with suspected cervical injury should not be allowed to sit, stand, or walk and should be lifted or rolled onto solid support boards. Gentle axial traction is used to support and maintain the head in neutral midline position during movement, and sandbags or hard collar should be used to help prevent lateral or flexion movements. In the emergency room high dose steroids may help diminish long-term deficits; methylpredinsone is used as a 30 mg/kg intravenous bolus followed by 5.4 mg/kg IV over 23 hours.

Two further conditions associated with various spinal injuries that may be present at the accident scene require immediate action. The first occurs with upper cervical cord injury where there may be partial paralysis of intercostal respirations or complete absence of respiratory effort. Immediate artificial respiration is required through standard cardiopulmonary resuscitation without neck hyperextension. Nasotracheal intubation by experienced hands under continued neck traction and minimal extension is ideal. The second condition is spinal shock from autonomic nervous system dysfunction, causing peripheral vasodilation, hypotension, and hypothermia. Even during transport, an effort should be made with two large bore IVs to rapidly infuse warm plasma or Ringer's lactate to maintain blood pressure. The patient should be kept covered and warm, often with a "space type" blanket while in the field. A urethral catheter should be used to relieve bladder distension.

If there is a neurological deficit or a demonstrable fracture with dislocation, skeletal traction should be instituted in the emergency room using tongs or a halo ring with appropriate weight and follow-up skull films. As with head injuries, blood should be drawn for hematological studies, blood chemistry, arterial blood gases, and blood typing. A Foley catheter should be inserted and 16 gauge IV lines begun.

Neurological evaluation can be expeditious. Its goal is to establish the degree and spinal cord level of injury. The major issue is whether the injury represents a complete functional transection of the spinal cord, producing a loss of all motor or sensory function below the level of injury. To establish this, the patient should be asked to move toes, feet, legs, hips, fingers, wrists, elbows, and shoulders against resistance. Strength is graded as 0 (no voluntary muscle contraction), 1 (flicker or trace of muscle contraction, no joint motion), 2 (active movement, but only with gravity eliminated), 3 (active movement against gravity but not against resistance), 4 (active movement against resistance), and 5 (full strength). Sensation is tested by touching with a pin over legs, arms, and perineum. Finally, reflexes are tested: ankle jerk, knee jerk, radioperiosteal, biceps, triceps, abdominal, cremasteric, and anal wink. A rectal exam is always performed. If the patient is comatose, muscle tone in the legs and spinal reflexes are evaluated for asymmetries.

Reflexes will be absent below the level of cord transection immediately after injury. Hyperactive reflexes can indicate an incomplete injury or cord contusion. Autonomic dysfunction distally will block sweating and vasomotor response as indicated by bladder/rectal tone and priapism. In the neck, C_6 controls wrist flexion, C_7 wrist and forearm extension, and C_8 finger movement; for sensation, C_6 innervates the thumb and index finger, C_7 long and ring fingers, and C_8 the small finger. In the back, L5 controls foot dorsiflexion and S1 foot plantar flexion.

In spinal cord injury there are several important syndromes to know: the complete cord syndrome, the anterior cord syndrome, the central cord syndrome, and a variety of partial cord syndromes. The *complete cord syndrome* is characterized by lack of voluntary movement and sensation in any modality anywhere below the level of the lesion. Systemic hypotension and depressant drugs can exacerbate this syndrome and should be excluded before declaring that the lesion is complete.

The *anterior cord syndrome* constitutes loss of movement bilaterally with preserved posterior column function. Although acute disc herniation can produce this syndrome, the cause is more often a vascular insult resulting from direct anterior trauma or anterior spinal artery occlusion. Its presence requires urgent radiological investigation to exclude disc rupture with compression.

The *central cord syndrome* occurs typically after a fall in the elderly. It is characterized by a loss of strength and sensation greater in the hands than in the legs, gait difficulty, and bladder incontinence. It usually does not require acute surgery and is associated with cervical spondylosis, which is an overgrowth of bone in the cervical canal.

Incomplete or *partial syndromes* are the most common and they involve a variety of asymmetrical motor and sensory losses. They all require investigation by CT scan and myelography or MRI to define the pathology and persistent areas of cord compression.

Cervical Spine Injury

Realignment is the major goal in the early management of cervical spine injury. This is especially true if the lesion is incomplete, so that management can preserve whatever sensory or motor function is still intact. Traction is the primary method of achieving realignment. This can be done on a Stryker frame with halo ring or cervical tongs, or in a motorized bed with a halo ring. Sequential lateral spine films are taken after increasing weights from 15–80 pounds over a period of 1–2 hours while administering muscle relaxants. If alignment cannot be established by traction alone and if good anesthesia and operative help are available, urgent surgery is indicated. This is especially true with bilateral jumped facets and an incomplete neurological deficit. Once alignment is achieved, it should be maintained either by continued traction or by placement of a fitted halo vest. Depending on the type of lesion, fusion surgery might be necessary.

Spinal shock is characterized by hypotension and warm extremities. It results from a loss of vascular tone due to autonomic injury and subsequent pooling of blood in the peripheral tissues of the body. It is best treated by volume replacement if the myocardium is strong, coupled with sympathomimetic drugs such as neosynephrine or dopamine, if neccessary.

Thoracolumbar Injury

Thoracolumbar injuries result from motor vehicle and sports accidents or from falls. Radiological evaluation is necessary in anyone with low- or mid-back pain after such an accident. These fractures are treacherous. They often do not produce significant leg weakness, and can lead to compression of the conus medullaris and cauda equina, resulting in bladder paralysis and sexual dysfunction. The first steps are evaluation, including neurological testing and CT scanning, and then stabilization with bone graft and instrumentation.

Acute Paraparesis or Quadriparesis

Paraparesis is bilateral leg weakness; quadriparesis invoves both arm and leg weakness. Spontaneous, rapidly progressive paresis is a neurosurgical emergency until a reversible cause is excluded. The important causes include acute disc herniation and epidural tumor (Table 5.2). A careful motor and sensory examination to ascertain the level of the lesion should be followed promptly by plain spine films and then by myelography or MRI. MRI is the method of choice if it can be done immediately. It gives satisfactory information about the cause of spinal cord compression without requiring a lumbar puncture, and in addition displays the direction and linear extent of compression as well as associated bony disease. If a myelogram is needed, it should initially be done with 2–3 cc of water soluble contrast injected into the lumbar space to ascertain whether there is a complete block. More dye may be added from above to obtain a view of the top of the lesion, and the site of the block should be noted. A normal myelogram excludes a surgically correctible lesion, except for the rare spinal arteriovenous malformation. Cerebrospinal fluid (CSF) from the myelogram should be sent to the laboratory for cell count, cytology, protein, sugar, VDRL, gamma globulin, oligoclonal bands, and culture. If pus is obtained, the likely diagnosis

Table 5.2. Causes of Acute Paresis

Cause	Treatment
spinal epidural abscess	surgical drainage
spinal tumor	surgical excision
spinal hematoma	surgical evacuation
trauma	realignment
"transverse myelitis"	medical management
viral (polio, herpes, rabies)	medical management
syphilitic or tuberculous inflammation	antibiotics
arachnoiditis	medical management
multiple sclerosis	medical management
postinfectious	medical management
necrotizing	medical management
Guillain-Barre	plasma exchange

is epidural abscess and laminectomy should proceed. If no CSF can be obtained from a lumbar puncture, consideration should be given to C_{1-2} puncture for dye insertion.

Acute Ataxia

Acute ataxia is a neurosurgical problem because of the possibility of a cerebellar mass as its cause. Headache, nausea, vomiting, and weakness of conjugate gaze to the side of the hematoma characterize this disorder. The CT scan is diagnostic with the appropriate window to separate bone from brain. If artifact obscures the posterior fossa, MRI may be done. Other causes of acute ataxia include cerebellar infarction, usually from occlusion of a posterior inferior cerebellar artery branch; acute labyrinthitis, associated with clinical findings of vertigo; and acute frontal lobe infarction. Infarction, especially in the posterior fossa, may also be an indication for surgery when there is cerebellar swelling and necrosis.

Management of acute ataxia includes careful assessment of the patient's state of alertness, limb coordination, gag reflex, swallowing, verbal articulation, and vital signs, especially heart rate. Walking must be tested in a patient with headache and nausea; if the gait is unsteady, imaging should be done immediately. CT scanning with special attention (thin cuts) to the posterior fossa or, still better,

MRI should be done. MRI can display the mass, its relation to the cerebellum and brainstem, and its nature without contamination by bony artifact. Evacuation of a lesion causing significant mass affect and ataxia should proceed expeditiously.

Coma

Plum and Posner define coma as "a state of unarousable psychological unresponsiveness in which the subject lies with eyes closed." Adams and Victor (1989) have separated its causes into three groups, as presented in Table 5.3.

Table 5.3. Causes of Coma and Their Diagnosis

Cause of Coma	Diagnostic Approach
1. Disorders with lateralizing findings	
a) epidural, subdural, or intracerebral hematoma	CT, no contrast
b) infarction	CT, no contrast
c) abscess	CT with contrast
d) tumor	CT with contrast
2. Disorders without focal findings	
a) metabolic disturbances	
1) diabetic acidosis or hypoglycemia	serum glucose, arterial blood gases
2) uremia	acetone
3) Addisonian crisis	BUN, cortisol
4) hepatic coma	SGOT, alk phosphatase
5) hypoxia	arterial gases
b) intoxication: alcohol, barbiturates	blood levels
c) seizure	history
d) trauma	history
e) infection: pneumonia, typhoid Waterhouse-Friederichsen syndrome	CBC and differential chest, PA and lateral
f) hyper- or hypothermia	body temperature
g) hypertensive encephalopathy	blood pressure
3. Disorders with coma and stiff neck	
a) meningitis	lumbar puncture
b) subarachnoid hemorrhage	CT scan
c) encephalitis	lumbar puncture

Establishing the Cause of Coma

On neurologic examination it is important to search for signs of brain stem dysfunction, asymmetry of neurological function, and meningeal irritation. A careful history should be elicited, including narcotic or other drug dose, precise mode of onset of coma, and any other illness. An emergency CT scan should be obtained while evaluating blood test results followed by a lumbar puncture if the CT reveals no mass.

Initial Management

If there is no surgically treatable lesion, ICU support with ventilation, nutrition, and bowel or bladder care should be arranged. Intracranial pressure monitoring should be considered if there is evidence of brain swelling on CT scan; cerebral perfusion pressure should be maintained above 50 mm Hg. One useful sequence for evaluation and resuscitation of the comatose patient is as follows:

1. Support airway, breathing, and circulation. In most cases intubation is necessary and should be done with as little neck manipulation as possible.
2. Evaluate temperature, pulse, blood pressure, respiration, neck stiffness, and neurological pattern.
3. Draw blood for blood bank sample, sugar, sodium, potassium, chloride, BUN, CBC, bleeding studies, ammonia, T4, and toxic screen.
4. Begin an IV line with isotonic fluid with dextrose.
5. Insert a Foley catheter and nasogastric tube.
6. Give 100 mg thiamine IV (for possible Wernicke's encephalopathy), 50 cc D50W (for hypoglycemia), and consider naloxone 0.4 mg IV (for narcotic overdosage).
7. Obtain an EKG and chest film and get cervical spine films if there is a history of trauma.
8. Obtain a CT scan.

Further management of the comatose patient is discussed under specific etiologies.

Status Epilepticus

Tonic-clonic status epilepticus occurs when repeated generalized seizures follow one another so rapidly that one seizure begins before the postictal period of the previous seizure ends. It is important to stop because of hypoxia and the effect of repeated seizures on the brain. Steps in management include the following:

1. Assure that the airway is secure, which often requires intubation.
2. Establish whether there is a history of epilepsy, drug ingestion, or head trauma, and draw blood for CBC, glucose, calcium, magnesium, sodium, anticonvulsant level, and toxic screen.
3. Give thiamine 100 mg IV followed by 1 mg/kg of D5W IV. Phenytoin (Dilantin) is the anticonvulsant of choice in adults, given intravenously in normal saline no faster than 50 mg/min to a total of 1,000 mg. Monitor EKG and blood pressure throughout its administration. In children, IV phenobarbital, 10 mg/kg is the first choice, being ready for intubation if necessary. In adults, phenobarbital 120 mg is the second choice if the patient is allergic to phenytoin or if phenytoin does not control seizures 15 minutes after its administration.
4. Lorazepam (Ativan), 1 mg bolus up to 2–4 mg IV may be a useful adjunct in stopping seizures that are disabling and require rapid action. Diazepam is less often used today because of its cardiac or respiratory depression. Other medications that may be useful are paraldehyde 5 percent in sterile saline as an IV drip up to 2.5 ml/kg or by rectal administration, and general anesthesia as a last resort.

Meningitis

Meningitis must be recognized promptly by the neurosurgeon both in the emergency room and in the postoperative period. Mental obtundation, headache, stiff neck, and photophobia are characteristic features. Subarachnoid hemorrhage, brain abscess, subdural empyema, and tonsillar herniation can mimic meningitis, particularly in the postoperative period when they may be masked by steroids.

A high index of suspicion must be maintained for meningitis in any patient who deteriorates after surgery, especially a child.

The definitive diagnostic procedure is a lumbar puncture. If a CT can be obtained easily, it should be done before the lumbar puncture in a patient with suspected meningitis. No more than an hour should be spent in obtaining a CT and it should be bypassed altogether if the patient is very sick but has no focal neurological signs. Gram stains and India ink preparation for cryptococcus should be done on all specimens from patients with suspected meningitis, along with aerobic and anaerobic cultures. The lumbar puncture results can be divided into one of three characteristic profiles outlined in Table 5.4. If the diagnosis of meningitis is made, prompt consultation with the infectious disease or medical service is indicated. Table 5.5 gives a rough guide to antibiotic management.

Table 5.4. Patterns of CSF Findings in Meningitis

"Purulent profile"
   (low sugar, high protein, and many polymorphonuclear cells)
   Causes: Bacterial meningitis
                    Early viral meningitis
                    Embolic infarction with endocarditis
                    Parameningeal infection
                    Early tuberculous meningitis
                    Acute hemorrhagic leukoencephalitis
                    Chemical meningitis
                    Behchet's disease

Lymphocytic low glucose profile
   (low sugar, high protein, and many lymphocytes)
   Causes: Tuberculous meningitis
                    Fungal meningitis
                    Partially treated bacterial meningitis
                    Viral meningitis
                    Carcinomatous meningitis
                    Sarcoidosis of meninges

Lymphocytic normal glucose profile
   (normal sugar, high protein, and many lymphocytes)
   Causes: Viral meningitis or encephalitis
                    Parameningeal infection
                    Bacterial meningitis
                    Partially resolving, parasitic, fungal or tuberculous meningitis
                    Guillain-Barre, postinfectious
                    Encephalomyelitis
                    Acute demyelinating disease

Table 5.5. Emergency Treatment of Meningitis

Age	Likely Origin	Antibiotic
Neonate (0–2 months)	B-streptococcus gram-negative	IV ampicillin 50 mg/kg bid, + gentamicin 2.5 mg/kg tid
Child (2 mo–20 yr)	H. influenzae N. meningitidis	IV ampicillin 300 mg/day in divided doses, plus chloramphenicol 50 mg/kg per day in divided doses. If penicillin allergy: vancomycin
Adult	pneumococcus	ampicillin 12 g/day, or penicillin 25 million u/day
Postoperative patient	S. aureus	oxacillin 12 g/day, plus gentamicin 5 mg/kg/day
Immunosuppressed		ticarcillin 200 mg/kg/day in 12 doses, plus gentamicin 5 mg/kg/day

Cardiac Arrest

Although cardiac arrest is not simply a neurosurgical emergency, it occurs often enough in neurosurgery to warrant presentation of crucial points.

1. Call for help and support ventilation and circulation by mouth to mouth respiration (14/minute) and closed chest massage (72 compressions/minute).
2. Use an Ambu bag with 100 percent oxygen and assisted ventilation and intubate when possible.
3. Clarify the events leading to the arrest while an EKG is done.
4. Begin an intravenous line and draw arterial blood gases.

Subsequent management proceeds as required by the circumstances of the arrest.

1. For ventricular fibrillation, defibrillate up to 360 joules, then give Lidocaine 1 mg/kg IV if defibrillation is unsuccessful.
2. In asystole, give epinephrine (1:10,000) 0.5 mg intravenously or intratracheally.
3. Bradycardia is treated with 0.5 mg IV boluses of atropine.

Suggestions for Further Reading

Adams RD and Victor M. *Principles of Neurology,* Fourth ed. New York: McGraw-Hill, 1989.

Eisenberg HM and Aldrich EF. Management of head injury. *Neurosurg. Clin. North Am.* 2:251–506, 1991.

North B and Reilly P. *Raised Intracranial Pressure: A Clinical Guide.* Oxford: Heinemann, 1990.

Plum F and Posner JB. *The Diagnosis of Stupor and Coma.* Third ed. Philadelphia: FA Davis, 1980.

Rea GL and Miller CA. *Spinal Trauma: Current Evaluation and Management.* Park Ridge, Ill.: American Association of Neurological Surgeons, 1993.

6

Neurosurgical Medications

It is increasingly important for the neurosurgeon to be aware of the indications and side effects of specific medications, including the limits of their approval by the Food and Drug Administration. Some of the most commonly used medications in neurosurgery are discussed in this chapter.

Corticosteroids

Corticosteroids have revolutionized the management of neurosurgical disorders that produce significant brain edema. Three are widely used: *dexamethasone, methylprednisolone,* and *prednisone.* Five mg of prednisone is equivalent to 0.75 mg dexamethasone, 4 mg of methylprednisolone, and 20 mg of hydrocortisone. (These are equivalent anti-inflammatory dosages but glucocorticoid and mineralocorticoid potencies are different.)

Steroids are used for brain tumors or abscesses with significant surrounding vasogenic edema. A recent study has demonstrated that high dose steroids also have a role in spinal cord trauma (Bracken et al., 1990). The literature does not clearly support their use in traumatic hematomas or closed head injury. Their use in small amounts as replacement agents in panhypopituitarism is life-sustaining.

A routine dosage for brain tumors is 4 mg dexamethasone 4 times a day or its equivalent. Adrenal suppression occurs in 1 to 4 weeks at this level and should be monitored carefully when steroids are withdrawn. The usual practice is to taper steroids by halving the dosage every 2 or 3 days.

The side effects of prolonged steroid dosage are numerous and can be very serious. These include metabolic, gastrointestinal, muscular, and psychiatric effects. Among the metabolic effects are diabetes mellitus sometimes requiring insulin, increased bone resorption with osteoporosis and aseptic necrosis of the femoral head and other joints, reactivation of tuberculosis and increased susceptibility to infection, and increased fat deposition in the abdomen and cheeks. One gastrointestinal effect is increased stomach acid production, which can be blocked by cimetidine or other selective histamine antagonists. Myopathy may affect proximal muscles, and acute psychological syndromes range from anxiety to psychosis.

Anticonvulsants

Neurosurgeons see many patients with brain tumors, trauma, or congenital anomalies who are on anticonvulsants. It is therefore important to be familiar with the actions and side effects of seizure medications.

Phenytoin (Dilantin) has traditionally been the drug of first choice for all seizures except those associated only with transient loss of awareness. Because of this drug's high frequency of adverse or allergic reactions, the neurosurgeon must be familiar with two alternative drugs, carbamazepine and phenobarbital.

Phenytoin has a plasma half-life of 12–36 hours. It must be given in normal saline to dissolve, and it can be given slowly (50 mg/min maximum for a total of 1 g) intravenously to achieve therapeutic levels in 30 minutes; cardiac arrest is one well documented side effect of rapid administration. Therapeutic levels of 10–20 ug/ml can also be achieved in adults over 4–6 hours if a loading oral dose of 1,000 mg is given, or over 24–30 hours if 300 mg is given every 8 hours for 1 day followed by 300 mg per day. Phenytoin should not be given intramuscularly because of poor absorption.

Commonly accepted side effects are gum hypertrophy and facial hair. A common allergic reaction to phenytoin is an itchy maculopapular rash that begins to subside within a week of stopping the drug. Toxic effects of phenytoin include ataxia, megaloblastic anemia, hypocalcemia, low protein bound iodine, osteoporosis, and fatigue. Allergic effects that are idiosyncratic include diarrhea, a "lupus-like" syndrome, and blood dyscrasias. Because of a small likelihood of cleft lip and other anomalies in infants whose mothers take phenytoin, many physicians change pregnant patients to phenobarbital; however it has not yet been conclusively established that Phenytoin produces such defects. Typical phenytoin dosages are 300 mg/day in adults, but the dose should be adjusted to maintain a therapeutic level of 10–20 ug/ml.

Carbamazepine (Tegretol) has a half-life of 9–15 hours given orally; it cannot be administered intravenously or intramuscularly. Its therapeutic level is 3–12 ug/ml. Toxic effects of carbamazepine include ataxia and fatigue or sedation. Idiosyncratic allergic effects are rash, severe leukopenia, and jaundice. Side effects are leukopenia of mild degree, drowsiness, gastrointestinal upset, and dry mouth. Carbamazepine is best used for tonic-clonic seizures as an alternative to phenytoin, and among some neurologists it is becoming the drug of first choice for such seizures.

Phenobarbital is the first choice anticonvulsant in young children and infants and the second choice in other patients who tolerate phenytoin poorly. Its main side effects are sedation in adults and rarely hyperirritability in children. As with phenytoin, monitoring of plasma levels is an important part of treatment. Phenobarbital can be given orally, intramuscularly, or intravenously; the usual dose is 60–180 mg per day either as one dose before bedtime or in three divided doses. Its half-life is 96 hours. Blood levels are aimed at 15–40 ug/ml.

Lorazepam (ativan) is used intravenously in status epilepticus to break seizures and has replaced diazepam as the drug of first choice. It has a half-life of 4 hours.

Diazepam (valium) has a half-life of 24 hours given orally and 1/2 to 4 hours given intravenously. It has been used in the past to stop status epilepticus but has lost favor today because of occasional cardiac arrest and respiratory depression associated with its use.

Valproic acid has a 16–18 hour half-life; its blood level should be 75–150 ug/ml. Significant liver toxicity is its main side effect. It is the drug of third choice for tonic clonic seizures.

There are several new drugs recently approved by the FDA; these include Vigabatrine. Felbamate has been withdrawn because of possible aplastic anemia.

Antibiotics

The initiation of proper antimicrobial therapy is essential to minimize the impact of infection in neurosurgical patients. Several antibiotics deserve special mention as they are important in the treatment of patients with neurosurgical disorders. The list of antibiotics from which to choose has expanded in recent years. This section provides a brief discussion of some of these agents that are most relevant to neurosurgeons.

Staphylococcus species are very often responsible for postoperative wound infections, shunt infections, and diskitis. Since over 80 percent of *S. aureus* strains encountered clinically produce penicillinase and thus are not inhibited by penicillin G, the penicillinase-resistant penicillins are central to the treatment of suspected or proven staphylococcus infections. *Oxacillin* and *Nafcillin* are useful drugs in this regard when intravenous therapy is needed. *Dicloxacillin* is a good oral agent.

Vancomycin is another useful agent, especially when methicillin-resistant *S. aureus* and *S. epidermidis* are encountered clinically. *S. epidermidis* is commonly a culprit in shunt infection, making vancomycin useful in the treatment of this problem. It is also important in the treatment of staphylococcal diskitis.

Cefazolin (Ancef), a first generation cephalosporin, remains a useful alternative in staphylococcus infections. It is often used in preoperative prophylaxis. Vancomycin and Nafcillin can also be used in the perioperative period as prophylaxis against gram-positive infection.

Osmotic Agents

The treatment of increased intracranial pressure is based on the manipulation of three compartments; CSF, blood volume, and brain. Omotic agents work by drawing water out of brain tissue and thus reducing the brain volume. Intravenous *mannitol* is the main osmotic agent used in neurosurgery. It is given as an intravenous bolus of 1 g/kg in a 20 percent solution for increased intracranial pressure. Its effects are seen in approximately 20 minutes. An alternative use is intermittent infusion of 20 g intravenously every 6–8 hours as needed to keep the measured plasma osmolarity in the 300–310 range. An indwelling Foley catheter is usually necessary. An alternative that is not as satisfactory in our experience is *glycerol* orally 1–2 g/kg every 6 hours. The plasma osmolarity must be carefully measured at least daily while using these agents.

Agents Affecting Blood Pressure

The most common cause of elevated blood pressure in the hospitalized patient is an exacerbation of essential hypertension. Sometimes blood pressure must be lowered acutely. Events when emergent anti-hypertensives may be needed include intracerebral hemorrhage, hypertensive encephalopathy, and brain stem manipulation at surgery. Three agents are particularly useful in these situations. *Nitroprusside* is administered in a mix of 50 mg/250 cc D_5W. Unfortunately, it tends to increase cerebral blood volume and therefore intracranial pressure. It can also cause cyanide toxicity. *Nitroglycerin* 30 mg/250 cc is especially useful in treating patients with cardiac disease. *Arfonad* has the direct effect of lowering vascular tone and hence blood pressure, but causes pupillary dilation and is therefore less useful. These agents are primarily used in treating acute hypertension. For longer-term blood pressure lowering, useful agents include *inderal*, the drug of first choice in smoothing out hypertensive peaks, and *hydralazine*, which can be given intramuscularly as well as orally but which has the problem of associated tachycardia and significant drowsiness.

Calcium channel blockers, used with success in cardiac disease, have been employed in the treatment of cerebral ischemia secondary to vasospasm. The mechanism of action involves the fact that elevated intracellular calcium (seen after ischemia) can result in cell membrane alterations and subsequent cell death. The primary neurosurgical indication for calcium channel blockers is the prevention of vasospasm secondary to subarachnoid hemorrhage. *Nimodipine*, a calcium channel blocker, has been useful in this regard when it is initiated within 4 days of the hemorrhage.

A variety of agents known as *hypertensive agents* are used to keep blood pressure elevated in the face of potential hypotension. If hypotension is secondary to hypovolemic shock, fluid and blood replacement is the appropriate therapy. If cardiogenic shock is the problem, agents such as *neosynephrine, dopamine,* and *phenyleph-*

rine are helpful as intravenous drips. These drugs should be used only in the intensive care unit with an arterial line and a CVP line in place. Patients in spinal shock often have some degree of hypotension and it is important to treat this quickly in order to maximize blood flow to the injured spinal cord. Low dose dopamine infusion is useful in this situation.

Sedatives, Analgesics, and Anti-inflammatory Agents

Sedation in neurosurgery is a double-edged sword. It enhances patient comfort, but can cloud the sensorium and alter the neurologic exam. Therefore, sedation should be used sparingly and agents with a short half-life are generally preferred. Commonly used sedatives include barbiturates, diazepam and other benzodiazepines, morphine, and major tranquilizers. For the young or middle-aged patient requiring mild sedation, *lorazepam* or a related compound is most useful. In a patient who requires immediate sedation, intravenous *sodium amobarbital* is effective, but intubation must be readily available since respirations can be depressed. An alternative is intravenous *morphine*. In the elderly agitated patient, *haloperidol* is a very useful drug given in 1 mg oral or intramuscular increments to achieve the desired sedation.

Analgesics are used perioperatively in neurosurgery and are commonly prescribed to patients with back and neck problems. One important group of analgesics are those that combine analgesic properties with anti-inflammatory actions. Side effects of these drugs can include gastrointestinal hemorrhage, nephro- and ototoxicity, and antiplatelet action. There are numerus medications in this category of nonsteroidal anti-inflammatory drugs (NSAID), but *Ibuprofen* is one of the most commonly used. It should be noted that *Acetaminophen* (Tylenol), another commonly used drug in these situations, is an analgesic, but has little anti-inflammatory action.

A second group of analgesics are the *narcotic cogeners*. These share the ability of having their actions reversed by naloxone. Their side effects include respiratory depression, constipation, pupillary narrowing, nausea, and postural hypotension. Tolerance (the requirement of increasing quantities to achieve the same effect) and addiction (a physiological and psychological craving for the drug) complicate their use. The Drug Enforcement Agency requires a careful record of these medications and has classified them from group I (Codeine, Darvon), which can be prescribed by telephone, to group IV, which requires very stringent controls. *Morphine* is the touchstone of these drugs: 10 mg of morphine is equivalent to 100 mg *meperidine* (Demerol), 130 mg *Codeine,* 60 mg *pentazocine* (Talwin), 10 mg of *Methadone,* or 2 mg of *hydromorphone* (Dilaudid).

Finally, some drugs are not primarily analgesics but have important analgesic uses. These include *Tegretol* for tic douloureux, *Lioresol* for flexor spasms, *Clonopin* for deafferentation pain, and *antidepressants* for pain associated with depression.

Suggestions for Further Reading

Allen GS, et al. Cerebral arterial spasm. A controlled trial of nimodipine in patients with subarachnoid hemorrhage. *N Engl J Med* 308:619–624, 1983.

Beers RF and Bassett EG. *Mechanisms of Pain and Analgesic Compounds.* New York: Raven Press, 1979.

Bracken MO, et al. A randomized, controlled trial of methylprednisolone or naloxone in the treatment of acute spinal cord injury: Results of the Second National Acute Spinal Cord Injury Study. *N Engl J Med* 322:1405–1411, 1990.

Samuels MA. *Manual of Neurology: Diagnosis and Therapy.* Fourth ed. Boston: Little, Brown, 1991.

7

Neurosurgical Procedures

Many atlases describe the specific techniques that are employed in neurosurgical operations. The intent of this chapter is to present a brief introduction to neurosurgical techniques without being exhaustive. Routine neurosurgical procedures will first be described along with several anesthetic considerations that are pertinent to neurosurgical patients; then emergency and bedside procedures will be outlined.

Routine Neurosurgical Procedures

Neurosurgery includes surgery on the brain, skull, spinal column, spinal cord, and peripheral nerves. Many factors contribute to the success of a neurosurgical procedure, including prompt and accurate diagnosis and excellent perioperative care. Good operative technique is another important factor which can certainly improve patient outcome. In this section the technical aspects of several routine neurosurgical procedures will be briefly outlined.

Craniotomy and Craniectomy

A craniotomy is a surgical opening of the skull in which the bone is removed and then replaced; a craniectomy is a craniotomy in which the bone is left out after it has been removed. Both are described by the part of the brain over which they open. A frontal craniotomy is made anywhere over the frontal lobe; pterional craniotomy over the frontotemporal region or pterion; temporal craniotomy over the temporal lobe (this is one area where the bone may not be replaced completely because of the protection offered the brain by the temporal muscle); parietal over the parietal lobe; suboccipital in the region over the cerebellum (another region where the bone is sometimes left out because of protection by the neck muscles); and parasagittal along the midline of the skull.

Cranial procedures may be divided into the opening, the management of the lesion, and the closing. The goal of the opening is to expose the abnormality efficiently and adequately while protecting surrounding brain. The bone flap should be just large enough to deal with the lesion. The goals of approaching particular lesions vary: for benign tumors, complete removal is the aim; for malignant tumors, wide internal decompression; for trauma, rapid removal of the lesion; for arteriovenous malformations, complete resection and clipping of arterial feeders; for aneurysms, clipping without injury to surrounding brain. In dealing with brain lesions important principals are the minimal retraction of brain tissue around the lesion and use of agents that dehydrate the brain to allow adequate space in which to operate. Important adjuncts are magnification, at least with loupes, and with the operating microscope for many lesions; and the use of the cavitron and the laser for tissue removal. An intimate knowledge of neuroanatomy is essential.

Good closure helps avoid postoperative complications. Important features are impeccable hemostasis, water-tight dural closure with pericranial or other graft if necessary, replacement of the bone flap, obliteration of paranasal sinuses with fat if they are violated, and closure of outer tissues in layers with particular attention to the galea.

Potential complications of cranial procedures include postoperative hemorrhage (1–2% of cases) and infection (1% rate except in trauma cases with contamination). Pulmonary embolism can also occur in the perioperative period (2%). Other complications depend on the particular type of lesion: the rate can vary from 1% to 15%. Mortality in elective craniotomy generally is 1–2%.

Carotid Endarterectomy

Carotid endarterectomy involves the removal of atherosclerotic plaques, thus increasing carotid blood flow. The procedure begins with anesthetic induction, which should be done with an arterial line in place and meticulous care to avoid hypotension and possible cardiac ischemia, since most patients have significant coronary artery disease. Electroencephalographic monitoring is used in many institutions to assess hemispheric ischemia; it should be started before the induction of anesthesia.

For the endarterectomy itself, a longitudinal incision along the sternocleidomastoid muscle is deepened by careful blunt and sharp dissection to the common carotid sheath. The artery is then gently dissected past the bifurcation into internal and external branches, blocking the carotid sinus with xylocaine. Pump tourniquets are loosely placed around internal and common carotid arteries in case a shunt is necessary. Some surgeons invariably use a shunt, others never do; our practice is to use it if the EEG flattens with cross clamping. After systemic heparinization, the internal, external, and common carotid arteries are clamped, an internal to common arterotomy is made from below the plaque to above it, and the plaque is cleaned off the arterial wall. The artery is closed after back flow is assured; often, a subcutaneous drain is used for 24 hours. Complications include silent carotid occlusion, emboli in about 3 percent of cases, cardiac ischemia in about 3 percent, and hemorrhage at the operative site in about 2 percent. The mortality rate is about 3 percent.

Trans-sphenoidal Surgery

Trans-sphenoidal surgery is the procedure of choice for most lesions of the sella turcica. The c-arm fluoroscope and operating microscope are important adjuncts, as is expert endocrine help in the pre- and postoperative phases. Broad spectrum antibiotics are used prophylactically, since access to the sella is achieved through the nose or mouth. The head can either be flexed slightly or the neck hyperextended; the semisitting position is most commonly used today. With an incision either under the upper lip or along the anterior nasal septum, the sphenoid sinus is entered and the anterior sella is drilled out. Curettes and pituitary rongeurs are used to remove the tumor. Complete removal is demonstrated by visualizing the diaphragm sellae. Closure usually involves a fat pad graft in the sella turcica.

Special complications include injury to optic apparatus or carotid artery, hemorrhage into tumor bed, and CSF leak; they occur in about 5 percent of cases overall. Incomplete resection occurs in

10 to 30 percent of cases in most series depending on tumor size. Mortality is less than 1 percent.

Stereotactic Surgery

Stereotactic procedures precisely localize a surgical instrument, an electrode, or radiation by means of calculated coordinates in three-dimensional space. These procedures include biopsies, craniotomies, and radiosurgery. They involve three steps: calculation of the lesion coordinates and entry site, placement of a burr hole access site, and performance of the actual procedure. The procedure is often done with the patient awake. In the new stereotactic frames, intubation is not usually a problem if general anesthesia is needed. The major problems are hemorrhage (about 1%) and unsatisfactory biopsy of tumor.

Two procedures, while not stereotactic in the strict sense, involve placement of electrodes or needles under radiographic control. Retrogasserian fifth nerve lesion-making for trigeminal neuralgia, either by radiofrequency or glycerol injection, is done using skull base landmarks with an electrode or needle placed in the cheek. Usually sedation is necessary for at least part of the procedure. Cordotomy, or incision into the spinal cord for chronic cancer pain, may also be done percutaneously using radiographic guidance.

Approaches to the Spine

The spine can be approached either anteriorly or posteriorly. The decision depends on the location of the pathology, the stability of the spine, and to some extent on the number of spinal segments involved. Generally, if the pathology is anterior, such as in a central cervical disc herniation, an anterior operation produces better results. If the pathology is posterior, or if multiple spinal segments are involved, a posterior approach is preferred.

Posterior Approaches

Laminectomy is removal of the laminae over the dorsum of the spinal canal. It may involve several laminae (a multiple-level laminectomy for spondylosis, spinal tumor, or infection), one side of the

laminae (a hemilaminectomy for unilateral disc herniation), or laminotomy (in which only part of one lamina is removed). Laminectomies are described by the segment and number of laminae involved—for example, a C3–C7 laminectomy extends from the third
cervical to seventh cervical laminae; a left L5 laminotomy is removal of the left part of the fifth lumbar lamina.

Indications for laminectomy include spinal cord compression
from bone overgrowth, ligament hypertrophy, epidural abscess, vascular malformation, and tumor. Laminectomy to relieve a markedly
compressive anterior disc rupture or tumor, especially in the thoracic region, may cause paralysis, presumably from the backward
buckling of the spinal cord into the laminectomy defect.

In some procedures, removing the lamina is the goal of the
surgery. In others, such as tumor removal or disc excision, it is
a prelude to the major part of the surgery. The decision as to the
number of laminae to be removed is an important one that should
be made before the operation begins. Intraoperatively, it is prudent
to identify the level by X-ray. Even more markedly than with craniotomy, the operating microscope has allowed safe removal of such
lesions as tumors and arteriovenous malformations of the spinal
cord.

Principles of spinal surgery include adequate exposure and meticulous hemostasis, minimal manipulation of the spinal cord itself
(for lateral tumors, therefore, working laterally and letting the cord
reexpand into the abnormal region), careful consideration of cord
blood flow (the artery of Adamciewicz, usually fed to the intercostal
at T6, should not be compromised; the hazard of the sitting position for cord flow should be remembered; and systemic hypotension should be avoided), water tight dural closure, and good hemostasis.

Because of its widespread use, disc excision deserves special
comment. In lumbar discectomy an important consideration is to be
certain the disc is the problem and not bony encroachment on the
foramen; CT through the affected area will help determine this. Microsurgical technique may permit the effective removal of disc material without a large laminectomy. If bony encroachment is part of
the problem, however, aggressive removal of bone is in order. Indications and complications of lumbar discectomy are presented in
another chapter. The major complications of lumbar discectomy are
failure to relieve pain, later reherniation, infection, CSF leak, and
injury to abdominal vessels.

A soft laterally extruded cervical disc can be removed in a posterior approach by performing a proximal foraminotomy over the nerve root and removing the disc from under the root. A complete laminectomy is not necessary for removal of a soft disc. Alternatively, anterior discectomy may be done as outlined below. For lateral or ventrolateral thoracic disc herniations, either a costotransversectomy (removal of the head of the rib and transverse process) or an approach through the pedicle is possible.

Anterior Approaches

Anterior approaches to the spinal column are increasingly popular because these approaches often provide the most direct access to the pathology. Therefore, a good rule for deciding whether to approach a lesion from the front or the back is that the approach be from the direction in which the pathology is located. In the cervical region, anterior discectomy has proven to be an effective procedure in the treatment of disc herniations. An intervertebral bone graft may or may not be placed, depending on the surgeon's preference; it has not been shown that grafting changes outcome. Graft may be taken from iliac crest or from donor bone. For cervical vertebral tumors, the entire vertebral body may be removed if accompanying stabilization is used; many metastatic tumors can be resected with great success in this way. In the thoracic and thoracolumbar region, anterior approaches are important for vertebral body fractures with cord compression as well as for some disc disorders. In the lumbar region, anterior approaches have generally not been as useful since most lumbar surgery can be done by reaching around the dural sac and because the retroperitoneal vessels present a major problem in the anterior approach.

For anterior cervical approaches, a horizontal or linear skin incision is followed by dissection medial to the carotid sheath toward the vertebral body midline, with special hand-held and self-retaining retractors to hold the esophagus and trachea medially. It is especially important to avoid injury to the esophagus. The correct disc level must be identified by X-ray. Adequate lighting and magnification, usually with the operating microscope, are necessary. Disc removal by curette and pituitary rongeurs is followed by careful attention to the posterior longitudinal ligament and any disc material behind it. There is controversy about whether to fuse the vertebral bodies after anterior discectomy; if fusion is done a piece of bone is taken from the iliac crest, or a dowel is placed. Complications of anterior cervical discectomy include infection, spinal cord injury, recurrent laryngeal nerve injury, tracheo-esophageal fistula, and damage to the vertebral arteries. For the anterior approach to the thoracic or thoracolumbar spine, a thoracic surgeon is an important ally for the opening.

Spinal Fusion and Instrumentation

Spinal fusions with or without instrumentation are performed for spinal column instability. Common causes of instability include trauma, tumor, and rheumatoid arthritis. Many instrumentation systems are now available for both the anterior and posterior spine. It should be remembered, however, that the role of instrumentation is to immobilize the involved spinal segments until bony fusion occurs. Without a successful bony fusion, all constructs will fail.

Peripheral Nerve Surgery

Peripheral nerve surgery requires knowledge of the anatomy of specific nerves. Important points are incisions that are cosmetically acceptable, exposure of enough nerve to get length if necessary, a suture line without tension if suturing is done, and a knowledge of the regeneration times and muscles of importance. These are discussed in Chapter 10.

CSF Shunts

Placement of a CSF shunt is often lifesaving if there is acute hydrocephalus. Either the ventricles or the lumbar subarachnoid space may be used as a source of fluid, and drainage may be into the peritoneum or the jugular vein. For ventriculoperitoneal shunting, a small catheter is placed in the ventricle, attached to a length of silastic tubing with a one-way valve, tunneled under the chest and abdominal skin, and inserted into the peritoneal cavity. For ventriculoatrial shunting the distal tubing is placed in the jugular vein. Correct positioning of the catheter in the superior vena cava just proximal to the right atrium is verified radiographically.

Neurosurgical Anesthesia

The goals of neurosurgical anesthesia are to provide satisfactory anesthesia and amnesia, to diminish intracranial pressure, to provide an optimum surgical field, and to allow the quickest possible postoperative recovery from anesthetic agents. The most useful anesthetic technique employed is intravenous phenobarbital 2–4 mg/kg for induction with maintenance by intravenous narcotics (fentanyl and morphine), coupled with nitrous oxide and hyperventilation to keep $PaCO_2$ 24–30 torr. These procedures avoid increased cerebral blood volume or flow and therefore do not increase intracranial pressure. Inhalation agents should be used infrequently; of those currently available, isofluorane is best because it diminishes cerebral metabolic rate. Both halothane and fluothane should be used sparingly. For intubation, careful preoxygenation is necessary: paralysis is achieved with succinyl choline 1–1.5 mg/kg or pancuronium 0.8 mg/kg.

Intravenous lasix 10–20 mg followed by mannitol 1 g/kg produces optimum operating conditions by decreasing the intra- and extracellular volumes within the cranial cavity. A Foley catheter should be placed before administering these agents because of the brisk diuresis induced.

Arterial blood pressure should be monitored continuously throughout any neurosurgical operation under anesthesia. To correct hypotension, neosynephrine is the agent of choice because of its relatively pure alpha agonist properties. Dopamine and aramine increase cardiac output and are therefore less satisfactory if increased intracranial pressure is a problem. Hypotension may be induced for long periods by increasing the amounts of inhalation agent; to treat acute hypertension either nitropresside or nitroglycerin given through a central line are preferred agents.

General problems in neuroanesthesia include air embolism, especially with the sitting position when venous pressure at the operative site may be negative, and cardiac instability. To detect air emboli, a precordial Doppler has the greatest sensitivity, but end-expiratory CO_2 monitoring or a pulmonary artery line provide greater specificity. Embolization produces decreased end-expiratory CO_2 and pulmonary artery wedge pressure. With brainstem manipulation cardiovascular instability can be a serious problem. Bradycardia may be treated with atropine .4 mg IV, and inderal in 1 mg increments may help tachycardia.

Emergency Neurosurgical Procedures

Ventricular Catheter Placement (Ventriculostomy)

Indications for emergency ventricular catheter placement include acute hydrocephalus after subarachnoid hemorrhage, traumatic intraventricular hemorrhage, and tumors obstructing the ventricular system. Acute hydrocephalus can present with a history of headache, vomiting, and obtundation. Physical findings can include drowsiness, papilledema, and quadriparesis. A CT scan determines the diagnosis. Bedside ventricular catheter placement is indicated if the patient is rapidly becoming less responsive or developing decorticate or decerebrate posturing.

An emergency sterile ventricular catheter set should be available containing the following items: sterile towels, scalpel handle and a #15 blade, 10-cc syringe and a 25-gauge needle, 2 cc of 1 percent xylocaine with epinephrine (1:100,000), 1/4" Hudson twist drill and bit, suction tubing and #7 suction tip, bipolar cautery tips and cord, curette, needle holder, 3–0 nylon suture, and ventricular catheter. Headlights, cautery box, and suction source should be available on short notice or kept in the unit where the ventriculostomy is being done.

The best site for twist drill placement is 3 cm to the right of midline and 10 cc behind the nasion in an adult or just behind the hairline in a child. Landmarks should be marked with the nose visible. The hair in the right frontal region is shaved as far back as the ear. The skin is prepped with betadine solution or alcohol, and 3–5 cc of 1 percent xylocaine with epinephrine (1:100,000) is injected at the stab site. A single stroke stab incision into the periosteum is made with the 15-blade scalpel. A twist drill hole is made slightly larger than the diameter of the ventricular catheter. The cautery is used to coagulate the dura; a spinal needle is a poor second choice and the twist drill a poor third. Vessels on the cortical surface are coagulated if they are in the intended path of the catheter. The ventricular catheter is then aimed at the medial canthus of the right eye and 1 cm in front of the tragus, and inserted to a depth of no more than 7 cm. If the ventricle is not tapped, a second pass aimed more medially and posteriorly is attempted, again stopping at 3 cm. If fluid is obtained it should not be allowed to escape. The proximal end of the catheter is tunneled a distance of at least 3 cm from the original stab wound and then connected to a sterile collecting system. The

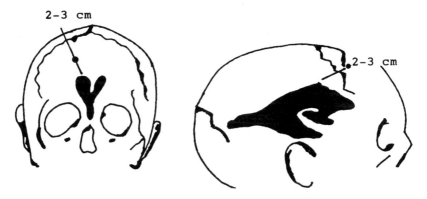

Figure 7.1. Approach to the lateral ventricle for emergency ventriculostomy.

catheter is sutured securely in place, checking intermittently to assure that flow continues once the catheter is finally secured. Instructions about the level of drainage and catheter care should be left with the nursing staff. Figure 7.1 illustrates this approach to the lateral ventricle.

Fiberoptic Intraparenchymal Transducer Placement

Use of a subarachnoid bolt to measure intracranial pressure is being supplanted by the use of nonfluid coupled devices, in particular a fiberoptic transducer, which is inserted 1 cm into the brain parenchyma. A small transducer is located at its tip. The fiberoptic transducer can be placed anywhere over the scalp not covered by muscle and away from the dural sinuses; the anterior frontal region over the side of the lesion is best for nursing care. A small twist drill is used and the transducer is inserted to a depth of 1 cm past the inner table of the skull. A calibrating screw is adjusted so that a zero reading is obtained on the amplifier. Visualization of a good waveform is necessary before one can trust the digital numeric display of ICP that is presented by the fiberoptic catheter tip transducer. The disposable fiberoptic catheter tip transducer has resolved many of the previous limitations of ICP measurement. Both fluid and tissue pressures are reliably measured with the same catheter. The catheter can be easily damaged, and is designed for use in a single patient.

Introduction of the intraparenchymal fiberoptic catheter tip transducer has been a significant advance in the continuous measurement of intracranial pressure. It is the state-of-the-art means of registering ICP in a comatose patient with intracranial hypertension; if it is not available, a subarachnoid bolt may be inserted.

Emergency Wound Reopening

It is occasionally necessary to reopen a wound in the recovery room or ICU if there is an acute hematoma in the operative site. This should only be done after discussion with the surgeon and as a last resort. A wound is usually reopened if deterioration is occurring so rapidly that there is not time for CT scanning or other studies. It should be done in the OR if time allows; if the patient is posturing or becoming paralyzed, the wound should be reopened in the ICU or recovery room. The skin is prepared with betadine and the wound is opened in layers with a sterile suture removal kit. If no extradural clot is found, the dura is examined; if it is bulging, it should be opened a little; if there is no clot the wound is packed with sterile sponges and the patient is taken either to the OR or, after rapid wound closure, to the CT scanner.

Epidural Hematoma Evacuation

The only case in which an epidural hematoma should be evacuated in the emergency room is that of the patient with a herniation syndrome who will die if more than 20 minutes go by without treating a clot. Hernation signs include progressive drowsiness or agitation, unilateral pupil dilation, and contralateral posturing. The following steps should only be undertaken if herniation is clearly occurring despite intravenous mannitol.

An available emergency kit should include linen, scalpel, syringe and needles, small self-retaining retractors, brace and bit, rongeur, curette, cautery, needle holder, suction catheter, #3 Penfield dissector, and bipolar cautery forceps.

If the site of the hematoma is unknown, surgery should be done at the site of a fracture if there is one, at the site of a major scalp bruise if there is one, or on the side of a dilating pupil if present. The hair is shaved and the scalp prepared with alcohol or betadine;

an assistant can do this while the surgeon opens the kit and puts on mask, gown, and gloves. One percent xylocaine is injected with 1:100,000 epinephrine into the skin. The temporal region is usually involved (middle meningeal artery) and care should be taken not to inject intra-arterially. A vertical linear incision is made 1 cm in front of the ear. Cautery should be used to get through muscle if possible, and the muscle is spread with a self-retaining retractor. Bleeding is stopped with cautery or clamp. The bone is opened with a perforator and the opening is enlarged to the size of a 50-cent piece with a rongeur. If no clot is found and the dura is tense, it is opened. If no clot bulges forth, the muscle is closed in one layer and the skin is closed tightly. A CT scan should be done as soon as possible to establish where the lesion is if one has not been found.

Placement of Gardner-Wells Tongs or Halo Ring

Tongs or the halo of a halo vest are important tools for aligning and stabilizing a spinal cord injury. To use Gardner-Wells tongs, a point 2–5 cm above the external auditory meatus is shaved bilaterally, prepared with betadine and infiltrated with xylocaine. The tongs are placed through stab wounds 3–4 cm above the external meatus; if flexion is desired, the tongs can be placed posteriorly to the line of the external canal. They have a spring-loaded pin in one screw that allows the force of application to be measured; usually 10–15 pounds is adequate (the spring pops out 1–2 mm). It is appropriate to begin with 10 pounds of traction in most cases. An alternative to tongs is a halo ring, placed 2 cm above the eyebrows.

Lumbar Puncture

A lumbar puncture is important to do as efficiently as possible, since problems introduced at the time of puncture may be difficult to sort out later. The major indication for lumbar puncture is meningitis. Contraindications include a unilateral intracranial mass with midline shift, a posterior fossa mass, or a lesion producing noncommunicating hydrocephalus.

The patient should lie close to the edge of the bed with legs flexed and back perpendicular to the bed. The lower lumbar region is prepared with antiseptic and xylocaine, and a wheal is raised between the spinous process of L4 and L5. A 22-gauge spinal needle is inserted in the midline pointing at the umbilicus. A pop is felt as the needle penetrates the dura: pressure should be measured immediately and fluid should be collected for cell count, protein, sugar, and culture if indicated.

Shunt Tap

For shunt tap, the scalp is shaved liberally around the reservoir of the shunt. A skull film is often useful in identifying where this is. The skin is prepared with betadine; petroleum jelly may be useful in plastering hair out of the way. A 23-gauge scalp vein needle penetrates the reservoir: fluid is collected for cell count, protein, sugar, and culture. The major risk is infection, making meticulous skin antisepsis important.

Suggestions for Further Reading

Fager CA. *Atlas of Spinal Surgery*. Philadelphia: Lea & Febiger, 1989.
Koos WT, Spetzler RF, Pendl G, et al. *Color Atlas of Microneurosurgery*. New York: Thieme-Stratton, 1985.
Ojemann RG, Heros RC, and Crowell RM. *Surgical Management of Cerebrovascular Disease*. Second ed. Baltimore: Williams and Wilkins, 1987.
Rengachary SS and Wilkins RH. *Neurosurgical Operative Atlas*. Baltimore: Williams & Wilkins, 1991 et seq.
Symon L, Thomas DGT, and Clark K. *Neurosurgery (Rob and Smith's Operative Surgery)*. Fourth ed. Boston: Butterworth, 1989.

8

Neurosurgical Management Procotols

This chapter summarizes pre- and post-operative care in neurosurgery.

Preoperative Care

A prerequisite for neurosurgical procedures in adults is obtaining normal preoperative bleeding studies (prothrombin time, partial thromboplastin time, platelet count). Electrolytes (sodium, potassium, chloride, carbon dioxide), BUN, and sugar should have been measured no more than 2 weeks before. The hematocrit should not be less than 38 in men or 33 in women without known cause; similarly, white blood count should not be above 10,000 wbc/min^3 without known cause. An electrocardiogram in patients over 40 or with known heart disease, a chest X-ray if none has been done within 5 years, and urinalysis complete the usual preoperative evaluation. A blood bank sample is usually necessary and blood should be set up if significant blood loss is anticipated (2 units is usually enough). In many cases today self-donation is possible. In otherwise healthy children, fewer laboratory tests are routinely ordered. Often, a urinalysis and hematocrit are sufficient.

On the day before surgery it is helpful to summarize laboratory data in a note that also describes the diagnosis and proposed procedure and documents consent. It is good practice to have a clear statement of what the defects are before surgery, with as much formal testing as possible to establish them .

Operative consent must be obtained before proceeding with any surgery and must be freely given and informed. The surgeon should describe the diagnosis, the possible procedures and alternative treatment methods to that proposed, the risks and complications of the proposed procedure, and its benefits. The choice of how much detail to provide must rest with the surgeon, but a cursory description is not adequate. Consent must be documented in some way in the record, whether by a brief statement by the surgeon, a written note signed by the patient, or a form signed by the patient and surgeon. It may be helpful to have a witness.

Certain problems can occur in obtaining informed consent. If a patient is incompetent (e.g., children, the demented elderly, or unconscious patients), the usual person to speak for him or her is the nearest relative, that is, the person who would give autopsy permission. In an emergency the best practice is usually to proceed with what is medically indicated if consent cannot be obtained immediately.

Special Preoperative Orders

Craniotomy and Craniectomy

Steroids are often used immediately before craniotomy, generally beginning 12 to 24 hours before. In patients at risk for seizures, anticonvulsants should be at therapeutic level before the procedure but may, if necessary, be administered intravenously just after the operation. Patients with infratentorial tumors usually do not need anticonvulsants. Preoperative antibiotics are used by many surgeons; they should be given intravenously no sooner than "on call" to the operating room and should be stopped 12 to 24 hours after surgery. The head should not be shaved more than 1 hour before surgery since new bacteria collect; a preoperative Hibiclens shampoo may help reduce postoperative infections.

Trans-sphenoidal Surgery

Endocrinological evaluation is important, as is formal neuro-ophthalmology testing if there is suprasellar expansion of tumor. Steroids should be given to protect the patient during the stress of neurosurgery.

Carotid Endarterectomy

Thorough cardiac evaluation is needed before surgery if there is any history of cardiac disease.

Laminectomy

Routine lab testing is usually sufficient.

Postoperative Care

General postoperative neurosurgical care includes careful observation by experienced nurses and house staff, control of blood pressure, and prevention of such postanesthetia complications as hypoventilation and atelectasis. This care can be divided into what is needed in the immediate 12 hours postoperatively and then subsequently. For the first 12 hours frequent checks of heart rate, blood pressure, respiration, level of alertness, wound region, and focal deficits should be made. Orders include:

1. General care: frequency of vital signs, diet, activity
2. Monitoring: arterial lines, fluid intake and urinary output, cardiac monitor if necessary
3. Drainage tubes: Foley catheter, CSF drain, wound drain if applicable
4. Postoperative lab tests: hematocrit, electrolytes, serum osmolarity, anticonvulsant levels, PT and PTT
5. Postoperative medication where applicable: intravenous maintenance, fluids, steroids, antacids, antibiotics, anticonvulsants, antihypertensives and blood pressure limits, analgesics, bowel medication, antipyretics, and antiemetics
6. Prophylaxis against venous thrombosis: pneumatic compression boots should be placed after induction of anesthesia and continued until the patient is ambulatory. Low dose heparin (5,000 u subcutaneously bid) may be started 24 hours following surgery in most cases.

Special Postoperative Orders

Craniotomy

For the first 12 hours postoperatively, the usual craniotomy patient is kept from having anything by mouth except ice chips. Hourly vital signs and neurological status are checked, intake and output are recorded, and the patient is on bedrest with the head elevated 30–45°. Steroids are administered and isotonic intravenous fluid is given at a slow (50 cc/min) rate. Mild analgesics such as acetaminophen are usually all that is necessary for pain; in fact, stronger analgesics are to be avoided because of interference with consciousness and neurological exam. For severe or labile hypertension a nitroprusside drip or nitroglycerin drip is used. Sublingual nifedipine, intravenous hydralazine, or intravenous labetolol are useful for milder hypertension. For acute hypotension, volume replacement with Ringer's lactate or human albumin is best along with a neosynephrine or dopamine drip. Great care should be taken not to overshoot and to be certain about why hypertension is occurring. After 12 hours, longer-term blood pressure control should be arranged if necessary. Steroids should be tapered off over a 1- to 2-week period.

Laminectomy

For 12 hours, vital signs are checked frequently depending on the risk of significant deterioration. A postoperative hematocrit after 12 hours is useful. Strong analgesics such as meperidine or morphine are often necessary and should be used liberally in the short term (e.g. meperidine 100 mg/3–4 h). Following lumbar or thoracic procedures where the spinal dura has been opened, the patient should be kept flat in bed for 1–5 days depending on the security of dural closure.

Trans-sphenoidal Surgery

During the first 12 hours, visual assessment is important with close monitoring of endocrine status as well. Hydrocortisone 100 mg iv every 8 hours may be used for the first 24 hours, starting just before surgery. This is tapered down to a maintenance dose of oral prednisone by the time of discharge. A morning serum cortisol should be checked before discharge to determine the need for long term glucocorticaid replacement.

Twelve to 24 hours postoperatively, patients may experience diabetes insipidus. This condition is diagnosed if the urine output is > 300 cc/hr with specific gravity < 1.003 while serum sodium is normal or elevated. Allowing the patient to drink freely is often sufficient treatment. Subcutaneous ddavp is given only if serum sodium rises above 150 or the patient is unable to keep up with fluid requirements.

Stereotactic Surgery

Gradual deterioration in the first 12 hours suggests hemorrhage and a CT scan is indicated. Deterioration over days suggests edema, and again a CT scan again should be carried out to confirm this.

Carotid Surgery

In the first 12 hours blood pressure control is crucial. Intravenous volume should be maintained, and the wound should be watched for hematoma.

Posterior Fossa Surgery

The patient must be watched particularly closely because of the possibility of brainstem compression and/or acute hydrocephalus with postoperative bleeding or brain swelling. Rapid deterioration mandates urgent wound reexploration.

Suggestions for Further Reading

Apuzzo MLJ. *Brain Surgery: Complication Avoidance and Management.* New York: Churchill Livingstone, 1993.

Haines SJ. Efficacy of antibiotic prophylaxis in clean neurosurgical operations. *Neurosurgery* 24:401–405, 1989.

Hamilton MG, Hull RD, and Pinco GF. Venous thromboembolism in neurosurgery and neurology patients: a review. *Neurosurgery* 34:280–296, 1994.

9

Neurosurgical Complications

Complications that the neurosurgeon must treat may be divided into those of a general nature and those that are specific for a particular procedure or disease.

General Complications

Atelectasis is the most common postoperative complication in neurosurgery. It is diagnosed in the presence of fever with diminished breath sounds or rales and sometimes diminished PO_2, most often on the first or second postoperative day. A chest X-ray may show diminished lung volume and platelike, high-density streaking. Early mobilization, avoidance of prolonged intubation in the postoperative period, and the use of incentive spirometry can prevent atelectasis or help treat it once it occurs. A particularly severe problem may develop if one mainstem bronchus (usually the right) was intubated during surgery; an entire lobe or lung may collapse, producing significant hypoxia. Vigorous physiotherapy and sometimes bronchoscopy and lavage are needed. If the patient remains intubated postoperatively, a positive end expiratory pressure (PEEP) of 5 mm Hg is recommended to prevent atelectasis.

Pulmonary embolism is the major nonneurosurgical cause of death in neurosurgical patients, with a 2–3 percent incidence of fatal outcome. Unfortunately, it can occur in young healthy patients with an otherwise good prognosis. Deep venous thrombosis is virtually always the source. Pulmonary embolism is best diagnosed by maintaining high clinical suspicion; fleeting chest pain or dyspnea should not be ignored and a ventilation/perfusion lung scan should be obtained readily. Treatment is heparinization and coumadinization for 6 months, or placement of an inferior vena cava filter. Sequential compression leg stockings are recommended to decrease the incidence of deep venous thrombosis and pulmonary emboli in nonambulatory patients as well as heparin 5,000 units subcutaneously twice a day to prevent the problem.

Pneumonia is clinically diagnosed by fever, hypoxia, and diminished breath sounds, and is definitively diagnosed by chest X-ray and sputum culture. The most common time of occurrence is 2–5 days after the operation. In a patient on steroids, fever may be absent, and the increase in white blood cell count minimal; in a dehydrated patient an infiltrate may not be evident. Treatment after obtaining sputum cultures includes not only an appropriate broad spectrum antibiotic, but also vigorous nursing care including positioning for drainage, chest percussion, and moisturizing the airway. After the specific organisms and their antibiotic sensitivities are identified, the most appropriate antibiotics are then chosen.

Pleural effusion can result from pulmonary cancer, infections, emboli, or heart failure. Medical consultation is helpful when an effusion of unknown cause occurs, and aspiration may be required to rule out infection.

Pneumothorax is a serious complication, especially if air can get into the pleural space but not out (tension pneumothorax). It may follow subclavian line placement. Dyspnea, diminished breath sounds on one side, and possibly tracheal deviation are characteristic and chest X-ray is diagnostic. If there is acute dyspnea, decreased breathing sounds, or tracheal deviation, a #18 needle should be inserted into the second intercostal space to relieve pneumothorax.

Respiratory arrest is a medical emergency requiring clearance of any obstructing material from the pharynx or trachea, ventilation, and cardiac massage until intubation is possible. Subsequent management is the same as for cardiac arrest.

Cardiac Complications

Myocardial infarction is sometimes obvious because of chest pain and hypotension. Hypotension alone or arryhthmia may announce it, however. The electrocardiogram is usually diagnostic, but medical advice should be sought in any case.

Cardiac arrhythmias manifest themselves as altered pulse rate or rhythm, acute dyspnea or palpitation subjectively, and EKG changes. Atrial flutter and fibrillation are treated with digoxin (or verapamil) intravenously or orally; elective cardioversion is necessary if cardiovascular insufficiency is significant. Ventricular tachycardia is treated with lidocaine and cardioversion.

Other General Complications

Gastrointestinal bleeding, manifested by hematemesis or melena, requires aggressive intravenous fluid replacement, blood replacement, gastric ice water lavage, and, if vigorous, placement of an intra-arterial catheter for vasopressin or somatostatin infusion. Gastroscopy is the definitive diagnostic step.

Agitation raises ICP and increases the likelihood that patients will extubate themselves. Catecholamine release consequent to head trauma may play a role in this agitation. Haldol and thorazine are effective agents. Ativan can also be effective, but has more sedative properties than the other two drugs.

Perforation of a viscus (bowel, stomach, appendix) is usually signaled by abdominal pain with tenderness, rigidity, and diminished bowel sounds on examination. In patients on steroids, these signs may be absent. An abdominal plain X-ray including an upright film or CT is necessary to establish the presence of free air, which establishes the diagnosis. *Intra-abdominal abscess* may occur after trauma or general sepsis. Signs include fever, pain, and tenderness; abdominal CT or ultrasound is the best diagnostic test.

Cranial Complications

Intracranial Hemorrhage

Hemorrhage may be into the brain parenchyma itself, the subdural space, or the epidural space. Progressive vomiting, drowsiness, hemiparesis, and other focal defects related to the site of bleeding are the major clinical findings. A CT scan is diagnostic and should be obtained on an emergency basis if hemorrhage is suspected. Particularly treacherous is hemorrhage in the posterior fossa, which may cause only headache, yet quickly progress to coma. Depending on location, mass effect, and physical findings, these hemorrhages could require emergent evacuation.

Seizure

The most likely cause of a postoperative seizure is a new hemorrhage. Phenytoin is the drug of choice unless the patient has an allergy to it. Benzodiazepines or phenobarbital may be given if urgent control is needed, with preparation for intubation and urgent CT scanning to assess why the seizure has occurred.

Infection

Intracranial infection may be epidural (an epidural abscess), subdural (a subdural empyema), intracerebral (an abscess), or in the CSF (meningitis). It is important to know that a patient with meningitis may have neither fever nor stiff neck if on steroids.

Pneumocephalus

Pneumocephalus occurs when air enters the head either after trauma or a neurosurgical procedure. It may be subdural, epidural, or intracerebral. Air acts as any other mass, and may produce serious disability if it is under pressure. A CT scan is diagnostic; treatment may include needle aspiration or sealing of a CSF leak.

CSF leak is important because of possible meningitis and/or intracranial air. Although small leaks may be watched for as long as 10 days, those persisting longer or profuse leaks will probably require repair. Frontal leaks may be repaired by fat obliteration of the frontal sinuses, and leaks from the mastoid region by fat obliteration of mastoid air cells. As a temporizing measure, a spinal catheter may help if there is no fear of pneumocephalus, which may occur when the intracranial pressure is lowered too much.

Unexpected Weakness or Other Focal Defect

If this is present when a patient awakens from anesthesia and is stable, think of an intraoperative stroke. If it occurs within 48 hours and is progressive, hemorrhage is more likely. CT scanning should be done in either case.

Brain Swelling

Cerebral edema occurs in certain circumstances for reasons that are still mysterious. It is especially problematic after operations on gliomas and meningiomas. Its management includes prolonged preoperative treatment with high-dose steroids (e.g., dexamethazone, 4 mg, orally 4 times a day), maintenance of high dose steroids postoperatively, dehydration with mannitol if there are significant clinical effects, and intubation and hyperventilation if necessary to preserve life. Large craniectomies are generally not helpful. The CT appearance of edema may be mimicked by early infection, especially cerebritis.

Spinal Complications

Paralysis

Paralysis is the most feared complication of spinal surgery. If it is present when the patient awakens from anesthesia, an obstructive cord lesion must be suspected. Has the graft slipped out of position? Is there a clot? Emergency spine X-rays should be ordered, and myelography or MRI may be necessary. CT scanning may not detect acute spinal hemorrhage. If no obstruction is found, the usual cause is a vascular spinal cord lesion. In the sitting position for cervical laminectomy, hypotension can lead to cord ischemia. During thoracic laminectomy, care should be taken to avoid the artery of Adamkiewicz, which enters between T4 and L2, often on the left, and supplies the entire lower spinal cord.

Spinal Instability

This is a later complication of extensive spinal surgery. It is rarely a problem in laminectomies when only the medial facet is removed. Realignment and fusion may be necessary if instability occurs.

Genitourinary Complications

Urinary tract infection is a mundane but potentially serious complication of catheterization. Important measures include removal of
the catheter as soon as possible, careful analysis of urine on withdrawal and vigorous treatment of any symptoms of urgency, burning, or frequency of urination.

Wound Complications

Subgaleal Effusion

This is a soft collection of fluid under a skin flap, which may result
from seepage of blood into the subgaleal space from stripped pericranial tissue or a dural leak of CSF. It is best left alone unless it
begins to compromise the skin edges, or leaks, or appears to be infected. It may take 3–4 weeks to resolve. If there is hydrocephalus,
it may not resolve and shunting either of the ventricles or sometimes
of the subgaleal space itself is necessary.

Wound Infection

This is manifested by a reddened wound with tenderness and fullness. Any collection usually requires drainage and removal of bone
flap, but intravenous antibiotics may be tried if the patient is closely
monitored and there is no palpable collection.

Complications of Positioning

Prone Position

Position shifts are avoided by making certain the head rest is tight
and pins are securely embedded. Avoid hyperflexion injuries of the
spine by appropriate positioning of the neck. Pad the iliac crest and
chest to prevent decubitus ulcers. Pulmonary emboli are avoided
with sequential pneumatic compression of the legs.

Sitting Position

Air emboli and hypotension are the most serious complications of the sitting position. Blood pressure must be maintained, usually by volume replacement, but also by vasoconstricting drugs; the arterial line should be at head level to be sure perfusion is adequate. Doppler or end-tidal CO_2 monitoring should be maintained to detect emboli early. The wound should be filled with saline and its edges packed with moist gauze if emboli occur, with gradual removal and cautery of possible offending vessels. The back of the head should be lowered if these measures do not work.

Suggestions for Further Reading

Apuzzo MLJ. *Brain Surgery: Complication Avoidance and Management.* New York: Churchill Livingston, 1993.

Chou SN and Erickson DL. Craniotomy infections. *Clin. Neurosurg.* 23:357–362, 1976.

Horowitz N and Rizzoli H. *Postoperative Complications of Intracranial Neurological Surgery.* Baltimore: Williams & Wilkins, 1982.

Wright RL. *Septic Complications of Neurosurgical Spinal Procedures.* Springfield, Ill.: Charles C. Thomas, 1970.

III

Neurosurgical Disorders

This section reviews the major pathologic processes encountered in neurosurgery. Each chapter will discuss these processes in terms of involvement of the brain, spinal cord, or peripheral nerves.

10

Trauma to the Head, Spine, and Peripheral Nerves

Head Trauma

The classification and triage of head injuries were discussed in Chapter 1. To briefly review, head injuries can be classified as mild, moderate, or severe according to the patient's symptoms. In mild head injury, the patient has a history of trauma but feels well except for such symptoms as headache, mild amnesia, or dizziness. Such a patient may be sent home with a "head sheet" if there is no focal neurological abnormality; when in doubt, a CT scan should be obtained. In moderate head injury the patient has focal findings or suggestions of increased intracranial pressure but can obey commands. In severe head injury the patient cannot obey commands.

Treatment of Severe Head Injuries

Medical Therapy

Approximately 40 percent of severe head injuries will require surgery; in the remaining 60 percent, medical management is the crucial modality. The major goals are control of intracranial pressure and prevention of seizures. Hyperventilation, lowering the $PaCo_2$ to 25–30 torr, can rapidly decrease intracranial pressure by causing cerebral vasoconstriction, thereby decreasing cerebral blood volume. Diuretics can decrease cerebral water content, intracranial volume, and ICP. A Foley catheter should be inserted before their use. Mannitol, in doses of 1–2 g/kg intravenously as rapidly as possible, increases serum osmolarity and draws free water from areas with an intact blood-brain barrier. A serum osmolarity of 300–310 mOsm/L is the desired therapeutic range; osmolarity greater than 320 mOsm/L can lead to irreversible renal damage. The effect of mannitol on ICP is usually evident in 20–30 minutes and lasts 4–6 hours. An exception to the general therapeutic effect of mannitol occurs in head injured children with evidence of hyperemic diffuse brain swelling. In these cases the increases in cerebral blood flow that follow mannitol administration may outweigh the diuretic effects, leading to increased ICP. Furosemide lowers ICP by decreasing cerebral blood volume and altering CSF production and absorption. Glycerol, urea and acetazolamide also can lower ICP but are used much less frequently than mannitol.

Corticosteroids have proven beneficial in the management of the cerebral vasogenic edema associated with brain tumors; there is no consensus in the literature, however, regarding their efficacy in the management of the cytotoxic edema induced by closed head injuries.

Anticonvulsants should be given prophylactically if there is CT evidence of contusion or hemorrhage. Phenytoin in doses calculated to achieve levels of 10–20 mcg/ml is the first choice; Tegretol or phenobarbital are other options. Nembutal is not a good anticonvulsant because of its short duration of action. Most ongoing convulsions can be controlled by the intravenous administration of 1 g phenytoin over approximately 30 minutes (no faster than 50 mg/minute); it must be administered in normal saline to avoid precipitation. Blood pressure and cardiac rhythm should be monitored closely during its administration. Intramuscular use is not recommended because of poor absorption.

Sedative or narcotic medication should be avoided in the head-injured patient so as not to complicate evaluation of the mental state. If sedation is necessary to perform a CT scan with minimum patient movement artifact, a short-acting barbiturate such as brevital or a short-acting narcotic such as fentanyl may be used with careful monitoring of respiration and blood pressure.

Surgical Therapy

Indications for surgery in head trauma include: 1) an open depressed skull fracture; 2) an intracranial hematoma with greater than 5 mm anatomical midline shift; and 3) a contusion associated with 5 mm or more of midline shift (unless it is in the primary motor or speech cortex or thalamus). The principles of surgery include an opening large enough to visualize and control bleeding points, careful hemostasis, and the use of medical therapy to control cytotoxic cerebral edema. Usually a large "question-mark" flap is the appropriate opening. In cases of underlying severe contusion and expected edema, leaving the bone flap out and closing the dura with pericranial or autologous dural graft to allow room for edema should be strongly considered. The bone flap can be preserved in the bone bank for replacement later.

Specific Injuries

Scalp Lacerations

Scalp lacerations frequently cause profuse bleeding. Hemorrhage is best controlled by placing 0 or 2-0 nylon sutures through the laceration including galea in a mattress suture. Hair around the wound should be shaved and the wound should be thoroughly irrigated prior to suture if bleeding allows this. Large lacerations are best closed with a two-layer closure, with absorbable sutures approximately at the galeal margins and nylon sutures for the skin edges.

A *cephalohematoma* is a collection of blood between the galea and the skull that is usually seen in children, often mistaken for a depressed fracture, and recognized by the fact that its boundaries are limited by galeal attachments at skull sutures. Observation is the best management with aspiration reserved for recurrent or persistent cases.

Skull Fractures

Simple or linear skull fractures may indicate serious injury to adjacent structures. Areas of particular concern are the temporal fossa with the middle meningeal artery; the occiput with a transverse sinus tear; and the midline at the vertex with a superior sagittal sinus tear. Patients with skull fractures should have a CT scan.

Depressed skull fractures can be diagnosed best by CT, although tangential skull X-rays may also be useful. Open depressed skull fractures require operative debridement, reduction, and inspection of underlying dura for laceration or hematoma. Depressions near dural sinuses can be particularly dangerous because the bone fragment can lead to sinus thrombosis, and bone fragment elevation may precipitate hemorrhage. Closed depressed fractures should be elevated if they are depressed past the inner table of the skull, especially if they occur over speech, motor, or visual cortex, if there is CT evidence of a dural tear, or if they are cosmetically unacceptable. In children, there is an increasing tendency to observe depressed fractures.

Basilar skull fractures are usually diagnosed clinically by hemotympanum, spinal fluid otorrhea or rhinorrhea, bilateral periorbital ecchymoses (racoon sign) or Battle's sign (superficial ecchymosis over the mastoid process that may develop up to 24 hours after injury). These fractures are difficult to demonstrate on plain skull films; the brow-up or verticosubmental view may demonstrate intracranial air or an air-fluid level in the sphenoid sinus that is suggestive evidence of basilar fracture.

Complications of basilar skull fractures include CSF leaks, hearing loss, and facial weakness. Occult CSF leaks may be brought to attention by the Dandy maneuver of tilting the head down in a sitting position to exacerbate the leak. Fluid drainage from the ear or nose can be definitively identified as CSF by detecting chloride concentration greater than serum; although glucose levels may be helpful as well, simple test tapes for glucose can be inaccurate. If fluid is mixed with blood, CSF will produce a halo ring around a drop placed on filter paper. Posttraumatic CSF leaks are usually self limited, stopping within 3 days. No attempt should be made to plug the leak with gauze, or other material, and no surgery is indicated for the first 10 days unless the leak is profuse. If leakage persists, serial lumbar punctures can be done or a lumbar drain inserted to decrease the subarachnoid pressure and promote closure. Antibiotics are usually not administered prophylactically since they can select hardier organisms for subsequent infection; however, close monitoring for meningitis should be maintained. Hearing may be impaired by petrous bone fractures, either through direct injury to the auditory apparatus or secondary to blood in the middle ear. Serial evaluations by an audiologist are occasionally necessary. The facial nerve may also be injured in petrous bone fractures; immediate peripheral facial nerve paralysis may indicate nerve transection whereas delayed onset of paresis suggests perineural swelling and carries a better prognosis for recovery.

Cerebral Shear Injury

Both experimental and clinical work indicates that the most common mechanism of closed head injury is a shearing of white matter axons. Careful experimental work in animals has demonstrated that differences in the angular velocity of impact and in rotational and translational components of force application may determine whether an injury results in hematoma formation or shearing of axons. The current belief is that the lesion that leads to coma with a normal CT scan is diffuse axonal shearing rather than brain stem injury. MRI scans have provided radiological evidence of shear injury even when CT scans are normal.

Cerebral Contusion and Hematomas

Cerebral contusions can be evaluated best by CT scanning; they usually affect the frontal and temporal poles where the brain encounters a rough inner skull surface. They characteristically produce intracranial hypertension several days after injury when swelling of adjacent brain is maximal. Management is the same as for any other traumatic intracranial mass lesion; if intracranial pressure cannot be controlled medically, the contused brain should be resected.

Intracerebral hematomas may result from cerebral contusions; occasionally the cause will be rupture of an aneurysm or an arteriovenous malformation that precedes head trauma. If there is a question of such a causative lesion, arteriography should be done; a CT or MRI with and without contrast may also be helpful as a screening test. Delayed hematoma formation after trauma is a well-described entity. Repeat CT scanning should be done in anyone who deteriorates neurologically after the original injury; in some series, the incidence of delayed hemorrhage is as high as 10 percent.

Epidural Hematomas

Epidural hematomas usually arise in the temporal region from tearing of the middle meningeal artery or elsewhere from lacerated dural sinuses, meningeal veins, or emissary veins. They have a characteristic lenticular shape that is produced as an expanding blood clot dissects the dura away from the inner table of the skull. The classic history is a blow to the head leading to a brief loss of consciousness from which the patient recovers (the lucid interval), only to experience headache, vomiting, loss of consciousness, hemiparesis and pupillary dilation. Many patients do not have this classic history, however. If brain stem compression is not reversed, cardiorespiratory arrest and death will ensue; rapid evacuation is crucial.

Acute Subdural Hematomas

Acute subdural hematomas result from lacerated cerebral cortical veins or arteries. There is often concomitant intrinsic brain injury such as contusion and laceration, caused by movement of the brain surface relative to the rough, rigid calvarium. The patient may be rendered immediately comatose. The lesion is easily diagnosed by CT scanning and requires rapid surgical evacuation. The mortality rate among patients with acute subdural hematomas is approximately 30 percent in patients who undergo surgery within the first 4 hours after trauma and 90 percent for those whose hematomas are removed after 4 hours.

Posterior Fossa Hematomas

Traumatic posterior fossa hematomas usually result from dural venous sinus injury by fractured occipital bone. Definitive diagnosis is possible by CT scan, but a third or fourth generation scanner may be necessary to avoid bone artifacts that can obscure a hematoma. Hematomas within the posterior fossa are particularly dangerous because of their propensity to compromise medullary cardiorespiratory centers and spinal fluid pathways; a patient may enter with only headache and suddenly die from irreversible respiratory arrest.

Gunshot Wounds

High velocity rifle bullets (over 700 meters/sec) cause greater damage than lower velocity handgun bullets (less than 400 meters/sec) generally responsible for civilian injuries. The bullet track is larger than the bullet diameter because of transmission of explosive energy to the surrounding brain; if the bullet passes through the head, the exit defect is usually larger than the entry wound.

Initial management includes rapid neurologic assessment, radiographic evaluation, and medical therapy to combat intracranial hypertension. Broad spectrum antibiotics are administered since the wound is "dirty." Plain skull films are useful because they are not subject to the "scatter" artifact that frequently obscures CT scanning, but a CT scan should be done as well to detect intracranial hematomas.

Surgical management of lower velocity gunshot wounds includes local debridement and hemostasis. Necrotic brain, bone fragments, and other debris should be removed. Deep bullet fragments are generally not probed for, as they are sterile; to exclude abscess, however, follow-up CT scans should be obtained. The prognosis of patients with gunshot wounds to the head is generally related to the patient's initial level of consciousness. Approximately 90 percent of patients who are alert on admission survive, though severely damaged brain tissue is subject to dangerous swelling or hemorrhage later.

Cerebral Vessels in Head Trauma

Cerebral blood vessels have a central place in the pathophysiology of head trauma. Torn meningeal arteries and venous sinuses may produce epidural hematomas; lacerated cortical veins and arteries may produce subdural hematomas. Aneurysms may rupture and cause brain damage as part of their hemorrhagic syndrome; penetrating wounds such as gunshot or knife wounds may cause pseudoaneurysms that later result in fatal hemorrhage. Finally, carotid dissection may cause neurological deficit secondary to injury from direct blows to the head and neck. The CT within the first 4–8 hours may not demonstrate any lesion in carotid occlusion; thus arteriography should be carried out in any patient with a severe localizing deficit and no apparent CT evidence to exclude carotid dissection or traumatic occlusion.

Late Sequellae of Head Injury

Post-concussion Syndrome and the Minor Head Injury

A minor head injury is sometimes as challenging to deal with as a major injury. Complaints of dizziness, headache, memory loss, fatigue, and nausea are common and appear to be physiological results of head injury rather than psychosomatic conditions or malingering. They should be treated symptomatically and are best followed by one person; prolonged time away from work may be necessary before they resolve.

Chronic Subdural Hematomas

Chronic subdural hematomas can occur after relatively minor head injuries, especially in the elderly. They develop over several weeks, usually leading to an initial complaint of headache with subsequent intellectual impairment and gait difficulty. Progressive enlargement occurs perhaps because of small episodes of rebleeding and osmotic effects. The physical examination may show a subtle hemiparesis, slight reflex asymmetry, and an extensor plantar response contralateral to the hematoma. The CT scan must be carefully interpreted and may require intravenous contrast infusion because the hematoma becomes isodense with the surrounding brain as blood reabsorbs. Contrast may show enhancement at the rim.

Surgical evacuation is indicated if there is significant neurologic deficit, midline shift, ventricular compression, progressive enlargement on CT, or rebleeding. Evacuation can be done at the bedside by inserting a closed catheter through a twist drill hole, or in the operating theater through burr holes. A full craniotomy is rarely necessary.

Posttraumatic Seizure

Seizures following mass lesions are common and can require long-term anticonvulsant treatment; their incidence is increased in patients with penetrating head wounds. They occur at two peaks, early and delayed (over a year after injury). There is debate over whether closed injury without contusion or hematoma should be treated with prophylactic anticonvulsants, but the policy in many centers is to administer phenytoin or another anticonvulsant for 6 months to a year after injury.

Post-traumatic Hydrocephalus

Ventricular enlargement following brain injury may be the result of brain atrophy or of a low-grade blockage to CSF flow; the decision to shunt is made by balancing the clinical symptoms against the risks of shunt insertion. A patient with arrested improvement or persistent gait difficulty and urinary incontinence who has ventricular enlargement should probably be shunted.

Spinal Cord Trauma

Serious injury to the spinal column may affect vertebral bodies, joints, ligaments, the spinal cord itself, or the nerve roots exiting from the spinal canal. The initial management and triage of spinal injuries was discussed on pages 72–75. There are three major questions to answer in approaching spinal injuries: 1) What is the level and extent of the injury to the spinal cord and nerve roots? 2) Is the injury reversible? 3) Is the bony spinal column unstable? The first two questions are answered best by neurological examination, the third by radiological studies and a reconstruction of the mechanism of injury.

Spinal Cord Syndromes

Several spinal cord syndromes have been recognized. They permit a classification of injury to the cord regardless of bony injury and an estimate of the lesion's reversibility. The most important initial distinction is between a complete lesion and an incomplete lesion. In a complete lesion, there is no voluntary motor or sensory response below the level of the lesion, and no bowel or bladder sensation. There is a patulous anus and complete perineal sensory loss. At first spinal shock prevents reflex activity as well as voluntary responses, but after several weeks reflexes may return. There is virtually no hope of recovery after a lesion has been complete for 72 hours with stable blood pressure, temperature, and metabolic state. Aggressive rehabilitation is the goal in these circumstances.

There are three generally recognized types of incomplete syndromes, though patients may have mixtures of them. It is more important to specify the neurological findings than to try to fit them into one of these categories.

The *anterior cord syndrome* is characterized by loss of movement, pain, and temperature sensation with retained touch, vibration, and position sense. The syndrome often results from compression or occlusion of the anterior spinal artery or of a major radicular artery. Its recognition warrants CT scanning, MRI, or myelography. If disc or bone is found compressing the cord, decompression should be carried out, usually from an anterior approach. The likelihood of recovery is small, however.

The *central cord syndrome* is characterized by greater motor and sensory loss in the hands and arms than in the legs. Urinary incontinence may occur as well. This syndrome occurs primarily in patients with extensive cervical spondylosis and is usually thought not to require surgery. Recovery of hand function is often incomplete. It is most commonly seen after trauma (often a mild hyperextension injury) in patients with underlying cervical stenosis.

In the *Brown-Sequard syndrome,* there is a loss of pain perception and movement below the lesion and loss of light touch, position sense, and vibration sense on the opposite side. This was initially described in a patient with a knife hemisection of the spinal cord and is rarely seen in a pure state. A more common partial lesion is variable motor loss with some sensory sparing. As with other incomplete syndromes, its significance is to suggest that further evaluation to decide on decompressing or realigning the canal is warranted.

Spinal shock is a syndrome characterized by hyporeflexia, hypotension, hypothermia, and either bradycardia or tachycardia. It may persist for 2 to 3 weeks in adults (much shorter time periods can be seen in children). In part it is a result of sympathectomy and consequent peripheral vasodilation. It can be treated with fluid volume and vasoconstricting medications such as neosynephrine or dopamine.

Cervical Spine Injuries

Possible injuries to the cervical spine include ligament tears, facet subluxation, fractures, and fracture-dislocations. They may be separated into those occurring with primarily a flexion mechanism and those that have a hyperextension mechanism. Axial loading is another common mechanism by which cervical fractures occur.

An important spinal injury sometimes overlooked in radiological examinations is tearing of ligaments, which may include interspinous ligaments, anterior and/or posterior longitudinal ligaments, and joint capsule. Usually these injuries will gradually resolve if only a small part of the ligament has been torn; however, they are an important cause of "whiplash" pain. If there is substantial tearing of interspinous and longitudinal ligaments, instability may result. At the time of injury, no bony injury may be evident and the patient's neck pain may limit movement; the only sign of injury may be widening between spinous processes in lateral cervical spine films. After 2 or 3 weeks, there is gradual slipping of one vertebral body on another because of ligamentous instability; the result is delayed spinal instability that can be a very serious problem. If it is recognized, the spine should be stabilized for 8–12 weeks in a halo vest. There is still a strong possibility that stabilization will not occur, however, and many surgeons favor elective operative fusion early when there is clear injury to ligaments.

Unilateral facet subluxations are common after a flexion-rotation injury such as that which occurs in diving. They may occur without associated spinal cord injury but more often are accompanied by severe neurological deficit, presumably from subluxation and partial relocation. The inferior facet of the upper vertebra slips up and over the superior facet of the lower vertebra. On anteroposterior views the spinous process of the superior vertebra is off midline; on the true lateral film the subluxed vertebra and those above it appear obliquely offset. An oblique film may show the disrupted joint. The CT scan is the best radiological test to demonstrate the overriding segment and perhaps a facet fracture as well. Unilateral facet subluxation is usually a stable injury, but it narrows the spinal canal diameter and compromises the foramen of the nerve root. In most cases it should be rectified by alignment using traction or, if necessary, surgical reduction. The exception to this policy is the case in which there are no symptoms; even here, however, and the likelihood of later joint arthritis and nerve root compromise, the narrowing of canal diameter argue for reduction.

The first step toward realignment is traction using Gardner-Wells tongs and up to 70 pounds of weight with careful radiological control to be certain that distraction between vertebral bodies is not occurring. This maneuver is often unsuccessful with unilateral facet dislocation because of fractures or soft tissue interposition; if it fails, there are several options. One is manipulation with turning of the head to facilitate facet relocation, a potentially hazardous maneuver. Another is to leave the joint subluxed. The third (and probably best option) is elective surgical reduction and fusion.

Bilateral facet subluxations are severe injuries that are usually accompanied by quadriparesis or quadriplegia; they indicate severe ligamentous injuries. On the lateral X-ray film there is marked anterior displacement of the affected vertebral body (often 50% or more). These injuries are unstable and markedly compromise the canal. Immediate realignment is crucial and should be done quickly using traction. These injuries require fusion because of the severe ligamentous disruption.

Fractures of the vertebral body may also accompany cervical flexion injuries. They range from teardrop fractures with a fragment of the anterior body pushed forward, to wedge compression fractures of the entire body. Careful attention should be paid to possible fragments pushed back into the spinal canal; CT will reveal these. These fractures do not often necessitate an operation, but require 10 weeks in a firm collar to heal. Fractures of the spinous process alone (clay shoveler's fracture) can usually be treated with a Philadelphia collar.

Hyperextension injuries are often associated with spinal cord injury even when there is no bony damage. This is particularly common in children and is known as SCIWORA—spinal cord injury without radiological abnormality. There may be a chip fracture of the anterior margin of the body inferiorly, providing a clue to the fact that an unstable injury has occurred.

Specific Cervical Fractures

Several upper cervical fractures have a characteristic X-ray appearance. The Jefferson fracture is a compressive and bursting fracture of C1 with lateral displacement of the lateral masses; it can be treated with a Philadelphia collar if total lateral mass displacement is less than 6.9 mm. Halo immobilization is needed for total lateral mass displacement greater than 6.9 mm. A hangman's fracture occurs bilaterally through the pedicles of C2, with the posterior arch of C2 remaining with the lower portion of the cervical spine. This is an unstable fracture that requires halo fixation. Fractures of the odontoid are classified as Type I (through the odontoid); Type II (through base of odontoid) or Type III (into body of atlas). Type I and III can be treated sucessfully with halo immobilization. Type II fractures will often require open fusion if displaced more than 6 mm.

Radiographic Evaluation of Cervical Injury

Radiographic studies of acute cervical spinal injury begin with a portable lateral cervical spine film, then a complete cervical spine series, and a CT scan if necessary. In evaluating the cervical spine series one should note the following points on the lateral view. Anterior to C2 the soft tissue in both adults and children should be less than 7 mm; anterior to C6 the distance from trachea to the anterior-inferior edge of C6 should be 16 mm or less in children and 22 mm or less in adults. The vertebral bodies need to be visualized down to the top of T1, and a "swimmer's view" may be necessary to accomplish this; more often a CT scan is done to evaluate this area. The vertebral bodies should be symmetrical, with a smoothly curving posterior border. The lateral facet joints should be superimposed on the body shadow; if they are not, unilateral subluxation is likely. Spinous processes should be equally spaced. On the AP open mouth view of the atlas, the base of the odontoid should be clearly seen. A cartilaginous line at its base in children less than 10 years old may be mistaken for a fracture. The lateral masses of the atlas should be equidistant from the odontoid and directly above the masses of C2 (the axis). Spinous processes should be in direct alignment. On oblique views, the neural foramina through which the nerve roots pass can be inspected for bone fragments. The laminae should overlap like shingles.

The CT scan is the single most useful study for evaluating the bony ring formed by vertebral body and laminae and for visualizing the fractures within it. The patient can be positioned without movement, and a scan is taken one vertebral body above and one below the fractured body. With 3 mm sections on a high resolution scanner, fractures anywhere in the bony ring can be assessed and subluxed facets can be diagnosed. Hematomas or disc ruptures are probably not reliably seen with CT. MRI provides better resolution of disc material.

Myelography is not useful in diagnosing acute spinal injury if there is marked bony displacement; it will show a block of the dye that can be predicted from the bony pattern. MRI is much more useful, showing compression of the spinal cord as well as bony displacement. If there is good bony alignment and the patient shows clinical worsening, or if the syndrome is an anterior spinal one, MRI should be done emergently to ascertain whether disc material is responsible for the problem. If MRI is not available, CT with subarachnoid contrast can be used to evaluate spinal block.

Definitive Management of Cervical Spine Injuries

Cervical spine injuries are managed by reduction to anatomical position and fixation by immobilization or operative fusion. To minimize spinal cord damage, reduction of cervical spine injuries should be done emergently, especially if the spinal syndrome is an incomplete one. The first step is insertion of tongs or the halo head ring. Tongs must be used with a Stryker frame but are easier to insert than a halo ring; the ring is especially useful if later halo vest placement will be the immobilization technique of choice. Weights, beginning with 10 pounds, are added in 10-pound increments every 15–20 minutes to a maximum of 70 pounds. Intravenous or intramuscular valium may promote relaxation. The addition of weights must be done in an X-ray unit where sequential films can be done. If there is no movement with 70 pounds, or if there is distraction without reduction, operative reduction and fixation will be necessary.

Surgery is indicated for the following problems in cervical spine injury: subluxation that cannot be reduced, acute disc herniation as documented by an anterior spinal syndrome with radiological evidence of herniation, and increasing spinal cord deficit with block.

Surgery should be done from the direction of the obstructing lesion. If facets require realignment, posterior exposure and intraoperative alignment of facets under direct vision in a halo vest or in traction on a Stryker frame is appropriate. If a vertebral body is wedged with bone or disc in the canal, the body or disc material should be removed from an anterior approach. Posterior fusion of C1 or C2 requires exposure of the occiput to C4 posteriorly. Potential dangers of surgery include changes in spinal cord blood flow leading to worsening neurological deficit and effects of physical manipulation on the spinal cord.

The major goal of definitive management of most spinal injuries is the maintenance of bony alignment. If this is done with traction in a Stryker or Roto-Rest bed, it requires 8–12 weeks of bedrest; this treatment is rarely used today. Early mobilization will prevent some of the side effects of prolonged bedrest; it can be carried out with a halo vest. In a halo, a patient can be sitting within a few days of the injury and can begin rehabilitation training. Similarly, if early fusion is carried out, mobilization can proceed quickly, often in a Philadelphia collar.

There is an increasing tendency today to mobilize patients as quickly as possible even with their injury. The management of acute (1–2 days) and subacute (3–10 days) spinal cord injuries should be carried out in a unit skilled at such management such as a regional spinal cord center. Features requiring special care in the subacute phase include respiratory status, nutrition, bowel and bladder management, deep venous thrombosis prevention, and skin care. Atelectasis is a major complication of immobility; frequent turning from side to side, deep breathing, and other physiotherapeutic maneuvers are important, and chest X-rays should be done early if there is fever. Nutrition is of great importance; oral nutrition must await recovery from ileus, common to cervical injuries, which may take several weeks. If ileus continues for over 5 days, peripheral hyperalimentation should be considered. A bowel regimen including stool softeners and glycerin or dulcolax suppositories every other day should be started early. Bladder infections are minimized by instituting an early straight catheterization regimen. Deep venous thrombosis in the legs can be prevented by subcutaneous heparin or external pneumatic compression. Meticulous skin care is mandatory to prevent development of decubitus ulcers and pressure sores.

Pharmacotherapy is limited in spinal trauma. High dose steroids have recently been shown to reduce disability from acute spinal cord injury. Methylprednisolone should be given as a 30 mg/kg IV bolus over 15 minutes, then 5.4 mg/kg IV over 23 hours. Antibiotics such as bactrim are important in the suppression of urinary tract infections. A regimen to suppress stomach acid is also important.

The long-term management of spine injuries consists of physiotherapy for strengthening of muscles partially lost, occupational therapy for learning to use muscles still available, long-term bowel and bladder care, and the use of extensive mechanical aids for increasing mobility despite quadriplegia. A patient with an injury at a level below C8 can become independently functional because of hand use; a patient with a C7 lesion may do so with great effort. Above C7 some institutional help is likely to be necessary. Overall the outlook for improvement in neurological function after severe trauma is bleak.

Thoracolumbar Injuries

Injuries at T10, T11, T12, and L1 are the second most common spinal injuries. They are important because of their subtlety and potential reversibility. The mechanism is usually a compressive force (e.g., jumping from a building or hitting the ground hard while tobogganing) or an automobile injury. A forceful automobile impact while wearing seatbelts may produce a flexion-distraction injury at the thoracolumbar junction. The mechanics underlying this injury include horizontal shearing of the ligaments and/or osseous elements at that level. A purely osseus injury is called a "Chance fracture" after a surgeon named Chance.

The clinical syndrome of thoracolumbar injury includes back pain and perineal numbness. It is vitally important to be aware of the possibility of conus compression in this injury. The patient may not complain of leg weakness but may have anesthesia of S1, S2, S3 and impaired bladder or sexual function. Perineal abnormalities should be assessed by careful pin testing of the perianal and genital region, by testing cremasteric and anal reflexes and rectal tone, and by bladder catheterization to assess overflow.

With these injuries, associated abdominal injuries are also important to exclude. X-rays should be taken of the entire spinal column as well as the region of interest because of the possibility of associated spinal injury. Plain X-rays usually show only a wedging of T11, T12, or L1 on the lateral view. Thoracolumbar injuries can be assessed best with CT or MRI; the typical pattern is disruption of the vertebral body with a large fragment pushed posteriorly into the spinal canal. There are often associated fractures of the spinous process and lamina, and the residual canal diameter is often significantly narrowed. Myelography is not helpful before reduction.

Therapeutic options for thoracolumbar fractures include surgical reduction and fixation or bedrest for 10–12 weeks. The appropriate choice depends on the patient, the surgeon, and the facility. Early surgery is probably the wisest course since prolonged bedrest can be difficult to tolerate. If the neurological deficit is increasing, surgery should be done. Thoracolumbar fractures do not usually require immediate decompression, especially if the cauda equina rather than conus is thought to be the source of symptoms. Observation for a period to assess spontaneous improvement is indicated in most cases.

The three surgical choices are laminectomy, a transpedicular approach, or anterior decompression. Laminectomy is the least desirable since the spinal cord can buckle backward through the laminectomy defect and may increase the deficit. Furthermore, laminectomy increases instability by destabilizing the posterior elements (the anterior elements are already unstable). The transpedicular approach accompanied by instrumentation and fusion provides effective decompression and stabilization. The anterior approach with removal of the vertebral body and intervertebral grafting is also a useful and important technique. Anterior instrumentation systems are available that provide immediate stability and obviate a posterior operation for placement of rods.

Lumbar and Sacral Fractures

Lumbar or sacral fractures are usually managed by bedrest. There is little indication for surgery unless there is instability or a persistent neurological deficit associated with marked narrowing of the canal or foramen by bone or disc, or unless there is an associated CSF leak requiring exploration. The posterior approach is used conventionally, because the spinal cord ends at the L1 level and is not in danger of injury here.

Gunshot Wounds to the Spine

Gunshot wounds and other penetrating injuries of the spinal column require careful evaluation and judgment. The first task is to assess the trajectory of the bullet, evaluating other injuries such as abdominal, thoracic, or cervical lacerations. In most cases debridement of the tract is indicated, but the bullet need not be removed unless it is copper jacketed. Only if there is a profuse CSF leak from the tract will laminectomy and dural grafting be necessary.

Acute Injuries to Peripheral Nerves

Three types of peripheral nervous system dysfunction are important in neurosurgery: acute injury, chronic entrapment syndromes, and peripheral nerve tumors. In dealing with the peripheral nervous system, an accurate knowledge of neuroanatomy is crucial.

In the upper extremity, the cervical roots C5-T1 form the brachial plexus. As the plexus begins it gives off the dorsal scapular nerves to the serratus anterior muscle (C5, 6, 7). A lesion that disrupts the plexus close to the cervical roots will cause scapular winging, a movement of the medial scapula away from the thorax; such a proximal lesion is unlikely to benefit from surgery. Horner's syndrome indicating sympathetic loss and elevation of the hemidiaphragm indicating phrenic nerve damage also suggest proximal and therefore irreversible injury. A cervical myelogram may confirm root avulsion by showing pseudomeningocele formation.

There are two common patterns of brachial plexus injury: an upper plexus injury, usually from direct downward pressure on the shoulder, and a lower plexus injury, from hyperabduction of the arm. The upper injury produces a weak arm and shoulder with a functioning hand, the lower a hand held in flexion with a strong arm. It is important to know the level of the lesion since injuries between clavicle and nerve root may warrant exploration, especially in an upper plexus disorder. The pattern of motor and sensory loss is the most helpful localizing sign. The general anatomy is that roots combine to form superior, middle, and inferior trunks. Each trunk bifurcates with an anterior and a posterior division, the former supplying flexor muscle groups, the latter extensors. These divisions subdivide into lateral, posterior, and medial cords, named by their relation to the brachial artery. Subsequently the cords divide into the peripheral nerves themselves (Fig. 10.1).

There are two major questions in brachial plexus injury: 1) What plexus elements are involved? This is established by the pattern of motor and sensory loss and by EMG studies. 2) Is the injury a neurapraxia (contusion of the nerve that may recover fully), axonotmesis (severing of the axon but contained continuity of the nerve sheath so that regeneration will occur), or neuronotmesis (division of the axon as well as nerve sheath) with little likelihood of recovery? This is evaluated by EMG studies and the passage of time. An expert electromyographer is of great help in the evaluation of plexus injuries. A 2-week waiting period is necessary before the EMG will show denervation potentials.

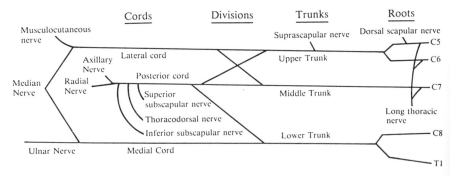

Figure 10.1. Schematic diagram of the brachial plexus.

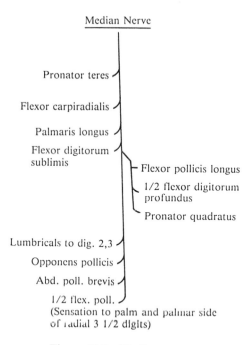

Figure 10.2. Median nerve.

The following general rules apply to brachial plexus repair with the likelihood of recovery: 1) If there is direct clean laceration, exploration in the first 2 or 3 days is warranted. If direct repair cannot be accomplished in that time, the nerve ends should be sutured to surrounding tissue to prevent retraction. 2) In dirty lacerations, traction injuries, or contusions, a waiting period of 6 weeks is warranted to assess whether there will be regeneration. Occasionally there is delayed deterioration from callous formation on clavicle or from an aneurysm of the axillary artery. This warrants exploration.

Injury to the major peripheral nerves (musculocutaneous, median, ulnar, radial) in the arm and forearm has a variable prognosis. In general, about 40 percent of the lesions will divide the nerve so that spontaneous regeneration will not be satisfactory. Again, knowledge of neuroanatomy is the crucial element in guiding evaluation and repair. Figures 10.2, 10.3, and 10.4 illustrate the courses and branches of the median, ulnar, and radial nerves in the arms.

The radial nerve is usually injured in direct trauma to the humerus. It should be explored in the midarm; chances of recovery of

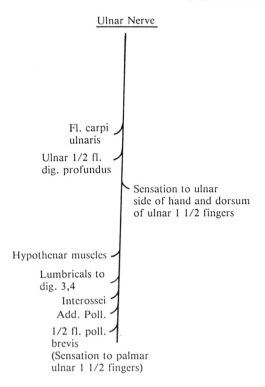

Figure 10.3. Ulnar nerve.

adequate motor function are excellent. The time for surgical repair is in the 6-week to 3-month period; after that satisfactory regeneration is unlikely. It is done either by direct suturing or by sural nerve grafting for greater gaps. Grafting principles include preparing the skin of the entire shoulder and arm to allow intraoperative assessment of muscle groups in the hand and forearm, using intraoperative nerve conduction studies to assess the continuity of nerves, cutting back the nerve edge to get fresh bleeding tissue, doing an anastomosis of perineurium to perineurium using interrupted fine silk suture without tension, and immobilizing the limb to allow optimal healing. Sutures are left in 14 days. If nerve repair is not satisfactory, the use of arthrodesis and tendon transplants to allow functional recovery despite irreversible neural loss is an important option and should be considered as part of the treatment plan by someone well-versed in upper extremity rehabilitation.

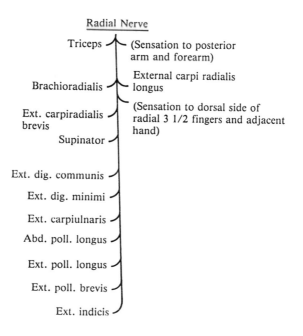

Figure 10.4. Radial nerve.

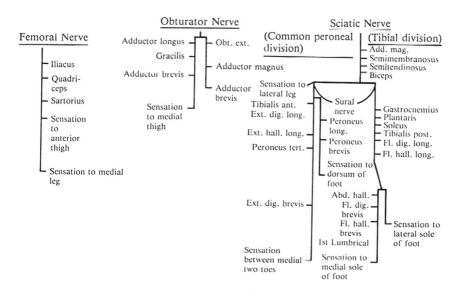

Figure 10.5. Innervation of the lower extremities.

The median nerve can be injured in the arm, forearm, or wrist. Loss of pronator teres muscle suggests an arm injury, loss of flexor profundi forearm, and loss of the flexor carpi radialis wrist. With surgical repair, some sensory improvement is likely but complete motor function is not.

The ulnar nerve is usually injured in the forearm. Its repair is unsatisfactory as reinervation of the multiple small hand muscle groups is incomplete.

In the lower extremities, the lumbar plexus has an arrangement similar to the brachial plexus; however its organization is not of the same direct clinical importance as that of the brachial plexus. Figure 10.5 provides details of its divisions: the femoral, obturator, and sciatic nerves.

Chronic Peripheral Nerve Compression Syndromes

Entrapment of peripheral nerves is an important problem that may be neurosurgically curable. In general, it is diagnosed by demonstrating a conduction block at the site of entrapment, usually indicative of focal demyelination. Common entrapment syndromes include carpal tunnel syndrome, ulnar nerve compression, and thoracic outlet syndrome.

Carpal Tunnel Syndrome

Carpal tunnel syndrome is the most common cause of hand or arm numbness in adults. It is characterized by numbness and tingling in one or both hands that may involve forearm and arm as well. Sensory loss is unusual on examination and often the only finding is weakening of the abductor pollicus. Median nerve conduction studies show prolonged distal latency with a block at the wrist; this is a requirement for diagnosis. The syndrome may be confused with cervical arthritis but the nerve conduction changes are diagnostic. If both conditions coexist, it seems prudent to treat the carpal tunnel syndrome first. Carpal tunnel syndrome is associated with states that increase soft tissue mass at joints such as pregnancy, trauma, rheumatoid arthritis, Paget's disease, osteoarthritis, myeloma, acromegaly, and hypothyroidism.

In treatment, temporizing measures such as injection of depo-medrol or wrist splints may be effective, but surgery is usually curative. Surgical release is done under local anesthesia with an incision along the mid-palmar crease and release of the flexor retinaculum with great care to divide the entire retinaculum and not to injure the recurrent motor nerves from the median nerve to the thenar muscles. Sutures are left in 10 days and patients should avoid heavy hand use for 6 weeks. The syndrome is cured in over 90 percent of cases; incomplete remission of symptoms is usually from incomplete retinaculum section or an error in diagnosis.

Ulnar Nerve Compression

The ulnar nerve is usually entrapped at the elbow, producing weakness of hand grip and numbness of the ring and fifth fingers. On examination there may be wasting of interossei and weak finger abduction. Either sensory or motor conduction, or both, may be impaired across the elbow on electrical testing. In 75 percent of cases the cause is unknown, although it may occur after an olecranon fracture (as "tardy ulnar palsy") or after direct compression at the elbow. It may be confused with cervical radiculopathy.

The first treatment is to eliminate recurrent compression by removing tight clothing bands or eliminating recurrent trauma. If symptoms are worsening, show no improvement 1 month after eliminating causal factors, or result from a compression that cannot be eliminated, surgery is indicated. Two procedures are commonly used: anterior transposition, in which the nerve is moved to a position anterior to the medial epicondyle and for best results embedded in the flexor origin; or medial epicondylectomy, in which the medial portion of the epicondyle is removed to allow the nerve to slide freely.

Thoracic Outlet Syndrome (Cervical Rib Syndrome)

This is probably overdiagnosed. It generally involves young adults with symptoms of hand and forearm tingling and usually weakness and wasting of ulnar and some median hand musculature. Results of EMG and nerve conduction studies are normal. X-rays show a rib or very large transverse process at C7. Vascular studies are nonspecific. Surgery is indicated only if there is muscle weakness or wasting: a supraclavicular incision allows sectioning of the scalenus anterior and resection of the rib or fibrous band producing the compression.

Other Compression Syndromes

Several other compression syndromes, though rare, are important to recognize. In the upper extremity, the *anterior interosseous syndrome* consists of weakness of index and long finger flexion with normal nerve conduction. The anterior interosseous nerve, a branch of the median nerve, should be explored if motor loss in flexor digitorum profundus and flexor pollicis longus is complete for 3 months. In the *pronator teres syndrome,* which consists of hand numbness and weakness in the entire median nerve distribution, the median nerve can be relieved by release of the ligament of Struthers or other compressive band. The *ulnar nerve* can be compressed in Guyon's canal causing hand weakness or numbness. Compression of the *posterior interosseous nerve* can produce wrist extensor weakness and requires exploration in the arm. The *suprascapular nerve,* compressed in the suprascapular notch, will cause selective pain and wasting of the supra- and infrascapular muscles. The *posterior tibial nerve* can be entrapped in the "tarsal tunnel," producing dysesthesias in the sole of the foot. The diagnosis is supported if injecting xylocaine yields relief. Surgical release of the flexor fibers will produce a good response.

Several nerves that are often involved in trauma or compression do not usually require surgery. Radial nerve palsies, caused by compression of the nerve against the humerus as in "Saturday night palsy," usually improve with time. A *hyperabduction syndrome* consists of paresthesias in the hands that simply repond to avoidance of hyperabduction. In the leg, *femoral nerve dysfunction* presents with quadriceps wasting, pain, and numbness in the anterior thigh, and loss of knee jerk. It is most often found in diabetics and rarely is helped by surgery. The *sciatic nerve,* which can be neuropathic with squatting or contusion, is rarely if ever entrapped; other causes must be sought for its spontaneous dysfunction.

The *lateral cutaneous nerve* in the thigh is often entrapped or injured but rarely requires surgery. The syndrome of "*meralgia pa-*

resthetica" with numbness, dull aching, and a burning of the antero-lateral thigh and diminished sensation is diagnostic. It can be distinguished from femoral neuropathy by lack of quadriceps wasting, extension of sensory loss to the anterior thigh, and preserved knee jerk. Similarly, it is distinguished from disc disease by the peripheral nerve pattern of sensory loss. If the paresthesias are intolerable, division of the fibrous band that overlies the lateral cutaneous nerve medial to the anterior superior iliac spine is usually corrective.

Compression of the *common peroneal nerve* produces foot drop with weakness of the tibialis anterior, peroneal, and extensor hallicus longus muscles. It can be distinguished from L4–5 disc rupture by the weakness of the tibialis posterior and hamstring muscles that accompanies the latter, along with back or radicular pain. It can be a part of Charcot-Marie-Tooth disease, in which case other findings and the family history are important. Diabetic peripheral neuropathy can also affect this nerve. In general, incomplete palsy as diagnosed by EMG or nerve conduction studies has a good prognosis. If there is progressive disability with nerve conduction block at the fibular head, exploration is warranted.

Suggestions for Further Reading

Cooper PR. *Management of Post-traumatic Spinal Instability.* Park Ridge, Ill.: American Association of Neurological Surgeons, 1990.

Dawson DM, Hallet M, and Millender LH. *Entrapment Neuropathies.* Second ed. Boston: Little, Brown, 1990.

Foulkes MA, and the Traumatic Coma Data Bank Investigators. Report on the traumatic coma data bank. *J. Neurosurg.* 75 (Suppl):S1–S66, 1991.

Levin HS, Eisenberg HM, and Benton AL. *Mild Head Injury.* New York: Oxford University Press, 1989.

11

Tumors of the Brain, Spine, and Peripheral Nerves

Brain Tumors

Brain tumors can be classified by histology as benign (meningiomas, vestibular schwannomas (acoustic neuromas), pituitary adenomas, craniopharyngiomas) or malignant (gliomas, astrocytomas, anaplastic astrocytomas, glioblastomas, oligodendrogliomas, ependymomas, metastatic tumors, medulloblastomas). Histologically, benign brain tumors may not be curable, however, because of their location; and some apparently malignant tumors like medulloblastoma have a significant survival rate. This chapter will deal with tumors by histological type.

Benign Brain Tumors

The most common benign brain tumors are meningiomas, acoustic neuromas, and pituitary tumors. Together they comprise 35 percent of all intracranial neoplasms.

Meningiomas arise from cells of the arachnoid membrane, which covers the brain; they may therefore be found anywhere in the brain or spinal cord. An important surgical point is that intact arachnoid surrounds the lesion, allowing a cleavage plane in most cases. The cause of meningiomas is unknown, though their increased occurrence in neurofibromatosis and their association with chromosome 22 deletion suggest a possible genetic predisposition.

Histologically benign meningiomas are classified as meningiotheliomatous, fibroblastic, or transitional depending on the predominant cell type. About 1 percent of meningiomas are malignant, and a variant called the angioblastic meningioma is very aggressive although it is histologically classified as benign.

The most common presentation of an intracranial meningioma is a seizure, either focal or generalized. Another common presentation is gradually increasing neurologic deficit. The character of the deficit depends on tumor location but may include hemiparesis, cortical sensory deficits, incoordination, or personality change. About 20 percent of meningiomas are parasagittal; they may produce unilateral or bilateral leg weakness if they are against the motor strip, or no symptoms at all if they are in the frontal or parietal region. Because they arise from the falx and involve the sagittal sinus, their complete removal is sometimes impossible. Convexity meningiomas (18%) produce symptoms referable to the cortex they compress. Subfrontal (17%) and sphenoid ridge (17%) meningiomas are often surprisingly large before symptoms appear. Parasellar meningiomas including those of the tuberculum sella (4%) and medial sphenoid ridge (6%) produce visual symptoms, especially visual field defects; their involvement with carotid artery, frontal bone, and cavernous sinus usually makes them only partially resectable. A variant that grows as a layer in the dura "en plaque" is similarly unresectable. Other less common meningiomas may have characteristic signs and symptoms: optic nerve sheath meningiomas present with monocular blindness, cerebellopontine angle meningiomas with hearing loss, spinal cord with spinal cord symptoms, and tentorial notch and intraventricular meningiomas may have almost no symptoms.

The CT scan, angiogram, and MRI complement each other in the radiological diagnosis of meningiomas. The CT scan shows a contrast-enhancing, hyperdense, homogenous mass with clearly demarcated smooth or lobulated contours and often reveals changes in the adjacent skull. The angiogram usually shows a vascular blush in the late venous phase; it may also demonstrate arterial supply from external carotid artery branches such as the middle meningeal or the artery to the falx. MRI usually displays increased signal on T_1 weighted images; with it angiography is usually not necessary.

The primary treatment for meningiomas is surgical excision. To be complete, excision should include the tumor, its dural attachments, and any involved bone; however, there is far from satisfactory ability to cure meningiomas by this method in some locations.

Convexity meningiomas can be removed in most cases; parasagittal tumors are more difficult because of sagittal sinus involvement. Subfrontal tumors can usually be completely removed, as can those of the cerebellopontine angle. Tumors that generally defy complete surgical excision are those of the medial sphenoid ridge, clivus, and tentorium.

Radiation therapy may be helpful in preventing recurrence of surgically unresectable meningiomas; overall, the 10-year recurrence rate in tumors with so-called complete resection is about 5 percent. If dura and bone are left, the rate is approximately 20 percent; if a significant part of the tumor is left, the rate is 40 percent. Despite these figures, the natural history of these tumors is that of slow enough growth to warrant incomplete resection if the danger of deficit with complete resection is over 10 percent and the patient is over age 50.

Acoustic neuromas (more properly called vestibular schwannomas) are benign tumors arising from the vestibular portion of the eighth nerve. They constitute about 5 percent of all brain tumors. Bilateral acoustic neuromas are associated with neurofibromatosis with a gene defect on chromosome 22. They arise from the Schwann cells surrounding the vestibular nerve and have two arrangements of cell types: Antoni A, in which cells palisade, and Antoni B, with a looser whirling arrangement of cells. They may become very large without producing more than hearing loss and some unsteadiness.

Hearing loss is an invariable symptom in these lesions, but it may be dismissed for many years as a result of aging or trauma. It is important to evaluate this early, as hearing can sometimes be preserved with small tumors and incomplete hearing loss preoperatively. Tinnitus and vertigo may accompany these tumors as well. Facial paresthesias and sensory loss accompany facial and trigeminal nerve compression by the tumor. With increasing size, cerebellar symptoms of unsteadiness of gait or limb and symptoms of hydrocephalus including headache and gait difficulty may follow.

The audiogram invariably shows sensorineural hearing loss in the affected ear. MRI is the imaging modality of choice. If gadolineum is injected intravenously, it will pick up lesions several mm in diameter. In distinguishing between the acoustic neuroma and less common neoplasms such as cerebellopontine angle meningiomas, CT of the internal auditory canal may be helpful; it will show erosion of the canal when there is an acoustic neuroma. Angiography is not useful.

Microsurgical excision of acoustic neuromas is presently the preferred treatment. The translabyrinthine approach has a lower incidence of facial nerve dysfunction than the retromastoid, but it invariably results in hearing loss and may not give adequate exposure with larger lesions. The retromastoid suboccipital craniectomy is the procedure of choice if hearing is to be preserved. Complete excision even of very large tumors can be accomplished by this approach. The improvement in surgical results over the last 20 years has been striking. These tumors now have a 1–2% mortality rate, with facial function preserved in over 80 percent of cases. For patients who have maintained some hearing in the affected hear preoperatively, there is about a 40 percent chance that it can be preserved if the tumors are less than 2 cm. In large tumors whose vascularity or brainstem attachment prevent resection, consideration can be given to radiation therapy. Stereotactic radiosurgery has been used recently as an alternative to surgery in some centers.

Pituitary adenomas have been found in as many as 25 percent of autopsies. They comprise about 15 percent of symptomatic brain tumors in surgical series. Virtually all pituitary tumors arise in the anterior pituitary (adenohypophysis); they have traditionally been classified according to the hormone-producing cells they contain. By immunoassay, pituitary tumors can be divided into prolactinomas (about 30%), growth-hormone producing adenomas (about 15%; some also produce prolactin), ACTH-producing adenomas (about 15%), glycoprotein-producing adenomas secreting LH, FSH, TSH, or the alpha subunit (about 20%), and tumors without apparent hormone products (about 20%).

There are two general clinical presentations of pituitary tumors: endocrine syndromes and syndromes of intracranial mass effect. Endocrine syndromes may reflect increased or decreased function. Five syndromes of increased function have been described with pituitary tumors. The most common accompany prolactinomas. In premenopausal women these are associated with amenorrhea and galactorrhea, in men impotence and rarely galactorrhea. Acromegaly, a disorder of growth hormone hypersecretion, is characterized by gigantism in children and adolescents and by broad chin and nose, prominent forehead, gap teeth, and wide phalanges of hands and feet in adults. More important than the skeletal changes in acromegaly are its metabolic abnormalities, which include cardiomyopathy and diabetes mellitus. Cushing's disease, caused by hypersecretion of cortisol from an ACTH-producing adenoma, is life-threatening;

truncal obesity, skin striae, capillary fragility, and buffalo hump are external features. The syndrome also includes diabetes mellitus, osteoporosis, and depression. Cushing's disease is the result of a pituitary adenoma; Cushing's syndrome is the same clinical picture from any cause including steroid therapy, or an ectopic source of ACTH. Nelson's syndrome is a disorder of ACTH overproduction in which prior surgical adrenalectomy has destroyed the adrenal cortex. It is characterized by skin hyperpigmentation and aggressive pituitary tumor behavior. Finally, there is a syndrome of overproduction of the alpha subunit. This occurs in both men and women with symptoms only of progressive loss of pituitary function.

In addition to syndromes of endocrine hypersecretion, there is also a syndrome of hypopituitarism that can be caused by large adenomas. Patients tend to be overweight with soft pale skin, loss of facial and body hair, and low energy. Men have small testes and women are amenorrheic.

The mass effects of a pituitary tumor are diverse. Headache is often felt at the top of the head, but has no particular distinguishing characteristics. Visual field loss from compression of the optic chiasm is usually bitemporal, but may also be unilateral. If the tumor extends into the third ventricle, obstructive hydrocephalus with headache, nausea, vomiting, and obtundation may result.

If it extends laterally into the cavernous sinus, extraocular palsies of the oculomotor, abducens, or trochlear nerves can be present. If it extends into the sphenoid sinus, nosebleeds may occur. About 1 percent of patients with tumor will present with pituitary apoplexy: this usually involves severe headache, nausea, vomiting, obtundation, and visual field loss or extraocular movement palsies from sudden tumor infarction, but less severe forms also occur.

Evaluation of pituitary adenomas includes radiological, endocrine, and ophthalmological assessment. On plain skull X-rays the sella turcica may be enlarged or asymmetrical; little else can be gained from them. CT may show a large tumor but bony artifact may obscure it. MRI is the imaging modality of choice. Small tumors may be detected within the gland and the full extent of larger lesions can be visualized. In sagittal reconstruction MRI will show a tumor's relation to the clivus and brainstem, and in coronal sections its relation to the optic chiasm.

Endocrine evaluation of a patient with a suspected pituitary tumor should include baseline prolactin, growth hormone, and 8 A.M.. cortisol levels as well as thyroid function tests. If these are normal, it may also be worth testing LH, FSH, and the alpha subunit levels since increasing numbers of apparently nonfunctioning adenomas appear to be associated with glycoprotein hormone production.

In evaluating prolactin, a level above 20 ng/ml is abnormal, but stalk compression effects can increase prolactin without a tumor. To be certain that a prolactin-producing tumor is present, the level should be over 200 ng/ml. To demonstrate growth hormone excess, a baseline fasting level greater than 10 ng/ml is diagnostic; failure of growth hormone secretion to suppress with hypoglycemia in an oral glucose tolerance test is helpful as well. To demonstrate overproduction of ACTH by a pituitary adenoma, two tests are necessary: first, documenting ACTH elevation by high fasting cortisol or 24-hour urinary corticosteroids; second, documenting that this high level is not suppressed by low dose (1 mg) dexamethasone given orally. ACTH production by an ectopic tumor may lead to high morning cortisol levels but there is no suppressibility by exogenous dexamethasone.

The treatment of pituitary tumors may involve medical, surgical, or radiation therapy. Medical treatment is most relevant in prolactinomas, where bromocriptine in increasing doses up to 30 mg a day may be used. The tumor will shrink and prolactin will return toward normal in 80 percent of cases; this usually occurs within a month of therapy. Major problems are nausea and the high cost of bromocriptine; furthermore, the neoplasm will usually regrow upon stopping this drug. CT or MRI scans should be used regularly to monitor diminution of tumor size. For other secretory or nonfunctioning pituitary tumors, medical treatment is limited although long-acting somatostatin analogues show promise in acromegaly.

Surgical therapy is very satisfactory for some pituitary tumors but not for others. There is some confusion in reporting "cure" rates; the present criterion for cure of prolactinomas is a serum prolactin less than 20 ng/ml; for GH-producing tumors, less than 5 ng/ml with normal dynamics; for ACTH-producing tumors, normal morning cortisol levels and low-dose dexamethasone suppressibility. By these criteria, microadenomas (tumors within the sella less than 10 mm in diameter) have a cure rate varying from 65 percent for prolactinomas to 80 percent for GH-producing and 90 percent for ACTH-producing tumors. Macroadenomas that are larger than 10 mm but entirely within the sella have similar results. Adenomas that extend outside the sella generally cannot be cured by surgery alone; their remission rate is in the 20–30 percent range.

There are still several challenging problems in pituitary surgery. With microadenomas, one of the most difficult may be finding the tumor. In Cushing's disease, radiographic studies may be normal, and exploration must be guided by endocrine testing. If no adenoma is found on exploration, several options are available; some surgeons recommend complete hypophysectomy, others partial resection of the gland most likely to harbor a tumor. For large pituitary tumors, problems include safe aggressive resection and adequate followup, which should continue for years.

Radiation therapy is a useful adjunct to surgery in pituitary adenomas. It reduces the recurrence rate at 10 years from 30 to 10 percent. There is, however, a small but definite incidence of postradiation panhypopituitarism. New techniques of focussed radiation including stereotactic radiosurgery and stereotactic radiation therapy are important adjuncts to surgery which minimize injury to surrounding brain.

The ideal therapeutic regimen still remains controversial; however, most authors would agree on the following. For prolactinomas that are microadenomas or intrasellar macroadenomas, bromocriptine is the first choice unless the patient wants to become pregnant or cannot tolerate the drug. In other cases of prolactinoma, surgery is the first choice. For acromegaly and Cushings disease, surgery is the first choice. Large tumors warrant surgery for two reasons: to decompress the visual system and to establish the histological tumor type.

Craniopharyngiomas have inspired disproportionate interest in the literature, perhaps because they challenge the neurosurgeon's skill to such a degree. They are histologically benign remnants of alimentary epithelium in the region of the hypothalamus. These remnants shed epithelial cells within them to increase slowly in size. Although histologically benign their location may make them act in a malignant way as they recur or continue to grow and compress the hypothalamus and visual apparatus. They are most commonly found in persons between 10 and 30 years of age but can occur at either extreme of life.

In adolescence or childhood these tumors present with delayed puberty, diabetes insipidus, or other pathological neuroendocrine states. Visual symptoms also occur early, clinically detectable field deficits being the most common manifestation. Skull X-rays show a normal or enlarged sella turcica. CT scans show an irregular, often cystic mass that may contain calcium arising from the sellar or suprasellar region. Detailed endocrine testing may demonstrate a variety of pituitary or hypothalamic deficiencies.

There is debate about how aggressive surgery should be in this condition. Many surgeons, however, feel that major resection which avoids injury to hypothalamus and optic chiasm, followed by radiation therapy, is the management of choice. New methods of focussed radiation therapy make this even more appealing.

Other Benign Brain Tumors

A variety of uncommon benign tumors are important to the neurosurgeon. *Colloid cysts* can occur in the third ventricle and lend themselves to complete excision. Their first presentation may be acute hydrocephalus or sudden death, especially if associated with hydrocephlaus. *Choroid plexus papillomas* are another cause of hydrocephalus and can often be totally removed. *Epidermoid* tumors occur most often at the skull base and are characterized by a lesion with lower density than CSF on CT; they may have spicules of air within them. Their border may be difficult to resect; the capsule should be removed as aggressively as possible but not pulled away vigorously from crucial structures.

Hemangioblastomas, vascular tumors that often have associated cysts, are important because they are usually resectable and because they are a feature of Von Hippel-Lindau disease with its associated renal cell carcinoma. They occur most often in the cerebellum and are characterized on CT scan or MRI by a low-density cyst with associated vascular nodule or by an enhancing mass. Resection of the vascular nodule will lead to complete cure of the cyst; failure to remove it will result in recurrence.

Epidermoid or dermoid tumors contain what appear to be desquamated fragments of epidermis within them. They are often clinically silent and are seen on CT as low absorption regions with CT values less than CSF because of the lipids they contain. Treatment is surgical resection in as much as is possible.

Arachnoid cysts are CSF-filled loculations lined by arachnoid cells. They occur in the temporal lobe, parasagittal region, or cerebellum, and may act as intracranial masses. If there is a progressive neurological deficit associated with them, excision or shunting may be indicated. Otherwise, they may be observed with sequential CT or MRI scans over many years.

Malignant Brain Tumors

Most malignant brain tumors arise from glial cells of the brain or as metastases from elsewhere. Gliomas, which include astrocytomas, glioblastomas, oligodendrogliomas, and ependymomas, are by far the largest group. Metastatic tumors comprise 10–15 percent of malignant brain tumors. Less common malignant tumors include medulloblastomas, sarcomas, and hemangiopericytomas.

Gliomas are thought to arise from glial cells, the supporting cells of the brain that are many times more numerous than neurons and, unlike neurons, can multiply after adult development. Glial cell types include astrocytes, which may have important nutritive functions for neurons; oligodendrocytes, which myelinate normal axons; and ependymal cells, which line the ventricular surface. Each has its own corresponding tumor type.

Astrocytomas are the most common primary brain tumor. Although their degree of malignancy varies, there are very few "benign" astrocytomas in terms of ultimate cure. In these tumors both the histological type and the location must be considered; apparently benign forms may nevertheless be incurable because of their location.

Most benign forms of astrocytoma occur in childhood. Potentially the most curable form is the cerebellar astrocytoma. This tumor causes dysmetria of arm or leg or gait difficulty with headache, vomiting, nausea, and other symptoms of diffusely increased intracranial pressure. Diagnosis is by CT or MRI showing a cystic cerebellar tumor without a hypervascular nodule. This tumor is treated by excision. Other low-grade childhood astrocytomas include optic gliomas, which occur in the optic nerve and chiasm, hypothalamic gliomas and spinomedullary astrocytomas. In children these neoplasms are characterized pathologically by Rosenthal fibers and only slight hypercellularity. Clinically, they have an indolent course in most cases. They produce symptoms referable to their locations: gradual visual loss for optic nerve gliomas; a syndrome characterized by emaciation, hyperactivity, precocious puberty, and hypotension for hypothalamic gliomas; and sensory or motor loss, often mild, for spinomedullary astrocytomas. The diagnoses are made by demonstrating symmetrical diffuse enlargement of the optic nerve and chiasm, hypothalamus, or medulla, respectively, by CT or MRI. MRI is especially valuable. Treatment is biopsy plus radiation, or, if the diagnosis can be made with very high probability, radiation without biopsy for optic and hypothalamic gliomas. Spinomedullary astrocytomas may be resected in experienced hands. Survival for many years is the rule, making it difficult to assess the efficiency of any particular treatment.

There are several grading schemes for astrocytomas. The most common is that of the World Health Organization, which divides them into astrocytomas (with hypercellularity), anaplastic astrocytomas (pleomorphism and hypervascularity), and glioblastoma multiforme (necrosis). A more recent scheme uses four criteria: hypercellularity, pleomorphism, vascular proliferation, and necrosis. Tumors with none of these are grade 1, with one grade 2, with two grade 3, and with three or four grade 4.

In young adults *diffuse astrocytoma* of the cerebral hemisphere may cause seizures or gradually progressive neurologic deficit. Characteristic locations are the frontal or subfrontal regions or the white matter of the hemisphere. The CT scan shows low absorption; an angiogram is of no use. MRI is the most valuable test for identifying these tumors and perhaps for establishing their extent; often regions that appear normal by CT will show up as quite abnormal by MRI. There is debate over appropriate management of these lesions. Generally, they are histologically low-grade and are often treated with whole brain radiation. Biopsy is important to determine histology, usually by stereotactic means if the region is otherwise inaccessible. Lobectomy is advocated by some surgeons if the region of the tumor is resectable.

Most adult astrocytomas are high-grade tumors of the cerebral hemisphere, also called malignant astrocytomas. They tend to spread far away from their origin, making their surgical removal impossible. They do not usually metastasize outside the CNS, although they may spread to the opposite hemisphere.

Anaplastic astrocytomas reach their peak in adults age 40–60, presenting with seizures, personality change, hemiparesis, sensory deficits, visual field loss, and other focal neurological deficits. Headache is not prominent. Treatment with chemotherapy and radiation prolongs median survival to 3–4 years.

It is not certain whether *glioblastoma multiforme* is different in origin or prognosis from anaplastic astrocytoma. These tumors are characterized radiographically by irregular enhancement with central necrosis and variable surrounding edema: the angiogram may show increased vascularity and early draining veins. The differential diagnosis includes abscess, infarct, and metastatic tumor. Pathologically they show necrosis, vascular proliferation, and nuclear pleomorphism. The natural history of these tumors is abysmal, with a life expectancy of 3–6 months without treatment. There is suggestive evidence that gross total resections are associated with longer survivals and improved quality of life. Treatment includes surgery to establish the diagnosis and remove as much tumor as possible followed by irradiation of 5,000–6,000 rads over 6 weeks. Attempts at chemotherapy have not been promising. Brachytherapy may have a role as it appears to lengthen life considerably. Given an aggressive program, patients with these tumors tend to have a satisfactory life-style until shortly before their demise 1–2 years after discovery of the tumor. Many neurosurgeons feel that such aggressive treatment is worthwhile.

Other members of the glioma family are less common: oligodendrogliomas are distinguished pathologically from astrocytomas by the "empty" appearance of their cytoplasm, looking like a fried egg. They have few of the highly malignant features of astrocytomas. They have a better prognosis than the malignant form of astrocytoma, with a mean survival of about 10 years, and are characterized on CT by calcification in a low absorption mass. Treatment usually consists of surgical resection and chemotherapy.

Ependymomas arise from the ventricular lining and are characterized by ciliary bodies on electron microscopy or ependymal rosettes histologically. They are most common in the fourth ventricle, invading its floor, and they occur primarily in young adults or children. They cause gait ataxia and hydrocephalus. Their treatment is resection as widely as possible followed by irradiation of both brain and spinal cord to prevent intraspinal "drop" metastases. Average survival is 2–3 years after discovery.

Metastatic Tumors

Metastatic tumors comprise 15–25 percent of brain tumors depending on whether the series is from surgery or autopsy. Hemiparesis, aphasia, seizures, and headache are common findings; these symptoms in a patient with a known malignancy should lead to CT scanning. The most common sites of origin of metastatic brain tumors are lung and breast. The differential diagnosis includes primary tumors and abscesses. On CT the mass is enhancing, with significant surrounding edema; there may or may not be central necrosis. The treatment is surgical extirpation followed by radiation therapy if the systemic disease and general medical condition warrant aggressive therapy. One-year survival is 50 percent on average; very often crippling neurological symptoms can be relieved completely with minimum morbidity using stereotactic techniques. Stereotactic radiosurgery has an important role as well, and may be used for selected multiple metastases as well as single.

Not uncommonly, metastatic cancer involves diffuse spread through the cranial and spinal subarachnoid spaces. This disorder, called meningeal carcinomatosis, is a particularly disheartening complication of cancer. It presents with signs of increased intracranial pressure including headache and papilledema, multiple lower cranial nerve deficits including facial and swallowing weakness, and arm or leg pain, any of which may be the principal characteristic. The pathological correlate is a sheet of tumor cells along the subarachnoid space ensheathing the cranial and spinal nerves. Tumors of breast and lung are particularly prone to have this complication, as are leukemias and lymphomas. The diagnosis is made by the clinical picture in the setting of known cancer and by lumbar puncture demonstrating increased malignant cells. The MRI scan may show increased enhancement especially in the tentorial notch. The natural history of meningeal carcinomatosis is miserable, and survival is virtually always less than 1 year. Combined cranial and spinal radiation therapy is the current treatment of choice.

Other Malignant Tumors

Medulloblastomas are important malignant neoplasms in children and young adults. In children aged 0–10 they present as midline cerebellar masses with truncal ataxia and subacute hydrocephalus. The differential diagnosis includes ependymoma and choroid plexus papilloma. In young adults aged 20–30 medulloblastomas occur more often in the cerebellar hemisphere, producing limb ataxia as a prominent syndrome. In either case the CT shows an enhancing mass of irregular contour, often with associated hydrocephalus. Treatment is surgical excision as completely as possible followed by radiation to the posterior fossa and spinal axis because this tumor is likely to have "drop" metastases. Chemotherapy has been increasingly used in the first 2 years of life. Overall prognosis varies, but over a third of patients now survive beyond 10 years and appear tumor free in adulthood. Sequelae of treatment have therefore become more important.

Germ cell tumors are a group of primary neoplasms arising from the pineal or hypothalamic region that have a confusing nomenclature and an embryonic relationship to gonadal tumors. They include dysgerminomas, teratomas, teratocarcinoma, embryonal cell carcinoma, and yolk sac tumor.

Primitive neuroectodermal tumors are histologically similar to medulloblastomas but occur in the supratentorial space. Their treatment is vigorous resection followed by radiation therapy.

Intracranial Tumors by Region

Because of their clinical manifestations and CT appearance, it is useful to consider brain tumors by their sites of growth as well as by their histological type. In the cerebral hemisphere, astrocytomas, oligodendrogliomas, metastatic tumors, and meningiomas are the most common neoplasms. In the cerebellum and posterior fossa, acoustic neuromas, meningiomas, epidermoids, and choroid plexus papillomas are generally found in the cerebellopontine angle; metastatic tumors, hemangioblastomas, medulloblastomas, and astrocytomas in children occur in the lateral cerebellar hemispheres. Medulloblastomas (arising from the roof of the fourth ventricle), ependymomas (arising from the floor of the fourth ventricle), and choroid plexus papillomas occur in the fourth ventricle and midline cerebellum. In the pineal region, pineoblastomas, pineocytomas, teratomas, and germ cell tumors are all possible but uncommon. In Japan tumors of this region are relatively common. In the suprasellar region, pituitary tumors, meningiomas, and craniopharyngiomas must be considered.

Spinal Tumors

Tumors of the spinal canal have traditionally been classified by their relation to the dura. Thus, spinal tumors are classified as extradural, intramedullary, or intradural extramedullary.

Extradural Tumors

Common extradural tumors include metastatic tumors, myeloma and lymphoma in adults, and neuroblastoma and lymphoma in children. Chordomas and sarcomas, including hemangiopericytomas, are also found extradurally, compressing the dural sac. They characteristically give an appearance of "feathering" around the mass and the dura can be seen as compressed from outside. Metastatic tumors are by far the most common extradural tumors; lung, breast, and prostate are the usual primary sites. Their treatment represents a difficult problem in neurosurgery.

Clinically, metastatic tumors to the spinal column may present with a known primary malignancy or de novo. Usually there is local back pain for months followed by gradually progressive weakness over several days. Typically the neurosurgeon is called when weakness is severe or there is complete paraplegia. The thoracic spine is by far the most common level, followed by cervical and lumbar segments. Plain X-rays may show destructive changes of bone; the pedicles, seen as "owl's eyes" on the AP view, are the most likely portions of the vertebra to be destroyed and their unilateral absence is a very important sign of metastatic bone disease. The vertebral body may be wedged in a partial fracture; its compression does not affect the disc space, a feature that distinguishes metastatic disease from infection. CT scans may show bony destruction not yet evident on plain films.

The sagittal views will demonstrate the extent of bony pathology, the nature of the compressive lesion(s), and the degree of cord compression. Transaxial views will show bony destruction, the relation of the lesion to the spinal cord, and the internal architecture of the compressive mass. Emergency MRI is an invaluable asset in assessing cord pathology.

If MRI is unavailable, CT may provide information about damage to bone but is not helpful in evaluating the cord outline. For this, the addition of an intrathecal water soluble contrast agent such as omnipaque is necessary and can be very helpful. Traditional myelography with dye placed above and below the block is a less good alternative.

Whatever imaging technique is used, it is important to move quickly once neurological deterioration is known to be occurring; a few hours may make a major difference. The primary question is whether radiation therapy or surgery should be used in the setting of neurological deficit and myelographic block. Although there is some disagreement, indications for surgery include a rapidly progressive neurologic deficit, lack of a known primary tumor and the need for a tissue sample, or a tumor that is insensitive to radiation such as a sarcoma. Judgment must be tempered by an estimate of the patient's longevity and general medical condition.

Surgery should be done from the direction that the tumor has grown, if possible. Simple laminectomy is often not the procedure of choice. In the thoracic or cervical spine with vertebral body destruction at a single level, anterior removal is indicated. Another option is to approach the spinal canal from posterolaterally, by drilling through the pedicle and into the body, then pushing the tumor forward into the space thus created. Using this kind of technique, some surgeons have demonstrated great success in improving neurological deficits from metastatic disease. Fusion may be necessary to restore spinal stability.

Metastatic disease to the spine raises several questions. One is whether to operate on a patient with known metastasis, spinal cord compression, and no neurological deficits. Some surgeons believe that radiation and close observation should be the initial management in such a case. However, others are now advocating a more aggressive approach consisting of anterior decompression. A second is whether to operate on a patient with progressive neurological deficit. This decision should be made in consultation with the oncologist, the patient, and the family, but our strong tendency is to recommend surgery. A third is whether to operate on a patient who has a complete lesion and complete block with no movement or sensation below the block. For practical purposes, the chances of any recovery from a lesion after it is complete (i.e., no movement or sensation) for 24 hours are so small as to make it most prudent to emphasize rehabilitation in this setting. If the interval since completeness is unknown or less than 24 hours, consideration may be given to surgery, but the chance of recovery is very small.

Intramedullary Tumors

Intramedullary tumors are important to identify as such because they may be surgically approached in many cases. They are the least common group of spinal tumors. They widen the cord contour on MRI or myelography. MRI is the procedure of choice in their diagnosis because it can delineate the structure of the cord itself rather than just the outline.

Common intramedullary tumors in both adults and children include astrocytomas and ependymomas. Epidermoid tumors may also occur in this location in children. Astrocytomas arise from the glial elements of the cord and present characteristically with increasing motor and sensory loss below the lesion. There is usually little pain. The cervical region is most commonly affected. On the MRI T1 weighted image there is a tapering long central cord mass with high signal intensity.

Traditional treatment has been biopsy through a laminectomy, followed by radiation. There has been an increasing tendency, however, toward total extirpation using the ultrasonic aspirator and monitoring with somatosensory evoked potentials. In children this appears to have remarkable success but should only be done in experienced hands.

Ependymomas arise from remnants of ependymal cells in the spinal central canal. They are more common in children than adults and occur either in the cervical canal or the conus medullaris. Every attempt at excision should be made for these and radiation may be added.

Epidermoids, dermoids, and hemangioblastomas may also occur within the spinal cord substance. Epidermoids may be rests of implanted cells from lumbar puncture; they are difficult to completely extirpate. Dermoids may be associated with sinus tracts to the skin; these tracts should be resected along with the tumor. Hemangioblastomas, which may accompany von Hippel-Lindau disease, may be totally resectable. Other ramifications of this disease, including renal cell carcinoma, should be sought.

Intradural Extramedullary Tumors

Tumors that lie within dura compressing the spinal cord or nerve roots are called intradural extramedullary neoplasms. They characteristically display "capping" with myelographic dye because of their direct contiguity with the subarachnoid space. These are often benign tumors and include neurofibromas, meningiomas, and lipomas.

Neurofibromas typically produce radicular pain with or without spinal cord compression in adults aged 30–50. Plain X-rays show enlargement of the neural foramen around the affected nerve root. The CT may show a lobulated mass that extends in a dumbbell shape outside the canal; this is clearly shown on MRI. Myelography displays a defect in the subarachnoid dye column. Treatment is microsurgical resection, which has a very good likelihood of cure. There is some ambiguity about the nomenclature of neurofibroma and Schwannoma. Most neurosurgeons use the term "Schwannoma" to refer to a diffuse neoplasm within the sheath of peripheral nerve or plexus, and "neurofibroma" to refer to a discrete mass in continuity with the nerve root but separate from it.

Intraspinal meningiomas occur most frequently in elderly women, presenting with pain, gradually progressive gait difficulty, and sensory loss. Treatment is resection.

In children, intraspinal lipomas are an important tumor in the conus region. They may be associated with a sinus tract. Their resection requires meticulous microsurgical technique.

There are several other rare causes of intradural extramedullary defects. Intracranial tumors such as medulloblastomas and ependymomas may produce "drop" metastases. Arachnoid cysts and neurenteric cysts, which probably have their origin in the embryological alimentary tract elements, may also occur in an intradural extramedullary location.

Peripheral Nerve Tumors

Peripheral nerve tumors are not common. There are four types: neurofibromas, Schwannomas, malignant neurofibromas, and metastatic tumors.

Neurofibromas are benign tumors arising from the Schwann cell nerve sheath and compressing the nerve without extending into its substance. They are usually completely resectable with contemporary microsurgical techniques. Occasionally their removal requires nerve resection and grafting depending on the preexisting nerve deficit, location of the lesion, and the patient's wishes.

Schwannomas are tumors that inextricably intertwine with the nerve sheath, nerve bundles, or fascicles, making their total removal without nerve division impossible. They are virtually always associated with von Recklinhausen's neurofibromatosis. Approximately 10 percent are malignant, in which case radiation therapy may be used as an adjunct to partial surgical removal.

Tumor metastases to peripheral nerve sheaths are uncommon; however, compression of peripheral nerves by tumor metastases does occur, especially in the lumbar plexus. Pain is a common symptom; it can be distinguished from the pain of disc disease by the absence of worsening with straight leg raising and general worsening when the patient is lying down.

Suggestions for Further Reading

Al-Mefty O. *Meningiomas*. New York: Raven Press, 1991.

Black P McL. Brain tumors. *N. Engl. J. Med.* 324:1471–1476, 1555–1564, 1991.

Burger PC, Scheithauer BW, and Vogel FS. *Surgical Pathology of the Nervous System and its Coverings*. Third ed. New York: Churchill Livingstone, 1990.

Kelly PJ. *Tumor Stereotaxis*. Philadelphia: W.B. Saunders, 1991.

Reed RJ and Harkin JC. *Tumors of the Peripheral Nervous System*. Washington, D.C.: Armed Forces Institute of Pathology, Supplement, Fascicle 3, Second Series, 1983.

Sundaresan N, Schmidek HH, Schiller AL, and Rosenthan DI. *Tumors of the Spine: Diagnosis and Clinical Management*. Philadelphia: W.B. Saunders, 1990.

12

Vascular Disorders
of the Brain and Spine

Strokes

A stroke is a neurological event of sudden onset resulting from disease in the blood vessels supplying the brain. Two broad categories can be defined: ischemic strokes, in which lack of blood supply leads to infarction; and hemorrhagic strokes, in which there is abnormal bleeding in the brain. There are three forms of ischemic stroke-thrombotic, embolic, and hypertensive, and two forms of hemorrhagic stroke- intracerebral and subarachnoid.

In the internal carotid system about 80 percent of strokes are ischemic; 35 percent are infarcts from carotid artery stenosis or thromboembolism, 20 percent are lacunes from small vessel thrombi, and 25 percent are embolic infarcts from the heart or elsewhere. The remaining 20 percent of strokes are hemorrhagic: 10 percent are intracerebral hemorrhages and 10 percent are subarachnoid hemorrhages. Brain tumors and seizures may mimic the stroke syndrome but can usually be distinguished by clinical presentation, EEG, and diagnostic imaging studies.

Strokes from Arterial Thrombosis

Thrombotic strokes can occur from occlusion of small, medium, or large arteries. In small vessels, hypertrophy of the artery wall from hypertension leads to occlusion. In medium vessels, emboli are the most common cause of occlusion. In large vessels, atheromatous narrowing produces occlusion and predisposes to distal embolization.

Small penetrating arteries to the basal ganglia, internal capsule, and thalamus may become thickened and suddenly occluded in a patient with systemic hypertension. The result is a small infarct that may or may not be visible on the CT scan but shows up as a small hole or "lacune" at autopsy. It is important to recognize lacunes clinically because they improve with time and do not require extensive investigation.

Lacunar strokes are small strokes in important areas. In general, their symptoms usually resolve in 48 hours, have stereotyped features, are maximal at onset, and present without headache or drowsiness. Certain patterns are characteristic: pure motor hemiparesis (weakness of face, arm and leg without sensory, speech, or visual loss), pure sensory stroke (numbness on one side of the body without motor findings), ataxia and crural paresis (unsteadiness and weakness of proximal legs), unilateral athetosis or other extrapyramidal symptoms, and dysarthria-clumsy hand syndrome. Multiple lacunes ("etat lacunaire") can lead to Parkinsonism, pseudobulbar palsy, and dementia.

The clinical syndrome of a lacune usually falls into one of the descriptions above. CT or MRI scanning should be done in all cases and angiography or Doppler carotid testing should be considered if the pattern is atypical or there is a cervical bruit. Repeat CT at 48 hours may show a lacune where none was seen initially, and MRI may show a lacune where the CT is normal.

Treatment of lacunes is primarily aimed at preventing further episodes. In the acute phase, blood pressure should not be lowered too quickly; for the long term, however, blood pressure control is the major therapy. Aspirin and other anticoagulants are not helpful.

Anterior, Middle and Posterior Cerebral Artery Strokes

Occlusion of these arteries is most often from emboli rather than from primary atherosclerosis, except in black Americans, who may have focal middle cerebral disease. The specific vessel involved can often be deduced from the stroke pattern. The middle cerebral artery has two divisions, upper and lower. An upper division stroke, involving the frontal lobe, will produce Broca's aphasia and hemiparesis in the dominant hemisphere; in the nondominant hemisphere, it will cause hemiparesis and hemineglect. A stroke in the lower division, supplying the posterior temporal and parietal lobes, will produce Wernicke's aphasia if it occurs in the dominant temporal lobe, and behavioral disorder if it occurs in the nondominant hemisphere. Main trunk occlusion will produce both disorders. Stroke in the anterior cerebral artery, supplying the medial hemisphere, leads to hemiparesis and sensory loss of the leg more than the arm. Because of the corpus callosum involvement, it may also produce left-sided tactile anomia (inability to name objects felt). Bilateral anterior cerebral infarcts produce akinetic mutism. Posterior cerebral artery infarcts have variable manifestations. With a unilateral infarct, there is contralateral homonymous hemianopia with macular sparing because the macula receives both middle and posterior artery supply; there may also be visual distortions or hallucinations. If the corpus callosum is damaged, there may be alexia without agraphia or aphasia. Bilateral posterior cerebral infarcts may produce cortical blindness with denial of visual loss, tunnel vision (only the macula preserved), or memory loss.

Carotid Artery Atherosclerosis

Carotid artery atherosclerosis occurs in a setting of generalized atherosclerosis, often accompanied by leg claudication and coronary artery disease. It can present either with emboli from atherosclerotic disease, or with hemodynamic slowing distal to a narrowed artery; often it is not clear which mechanism is operative. Carotid disease is characterized by a fluctuating course for days, weeks, and months, with variable attacks of eye or hemisphere symptomatology. In the eyes, transient monocular blindness or "amaurosis fugax" occurs; this is episodic unilateral visual loss "as if a shade was lowered," lasting for minutes to hours. In the hemisphere, episodes of aphasia, limb tingling, or weakness are characteristic. These episodes have been classified by their temporal course and reversibility. If they last less than 24 hours, they are called transient ischemic attacks (TIAs) and are generally thought to be from microemboli. If they last more than 24 hours but resolve completely within 3 weeks, they are called reversible ischemic neurological deficits (RINDs). If they are irreversible they are considered infarcts. Finally, there is an entity known as "progressive stroke" or "stroke in evolution," characterized by gradually increasing deficit in an area of low flow.

Physical signs may be helpful in establishing the carotid artery as the source of stroke. There is usually a carotid bruit, although recent carotid occlusion may present without one. A focal high-pitched bruit that lasts most of the cardiac cycle is characteristic of tight stenosis. Palpation of the carotid is of little use. Ophthalmic examination may show a Horner's syndrome and retinal infarcts or microemboli. Peripheral pulses may be diminished.

A variety of so-called noninvasive tests can be used to determine the hemodynamic significance of a bruit and the residual lumen of the carotid artery; in conjunction with an arteriogram, they help to establish the fact that a stenosis is slowing flow. These tests include oculoplethysmography, doppler imaging, thermography, palpation of facial pulses, and phonoangiography. A battery of tests may give maximum information, but Doppler ultrasonography is particularly well developed.

The transfemoral contrast angiogram is the most reliable test for evaluating the carotid artery. It is best done with transfemoral catheterization by a radiologist or neurosurgeon familiar with this technique. In experienced hands morbidity should be less than 2 percent even with carotid stenosis. Digital subtraction angiography, a technique ordinarily used with intravenous injection of dye, is not adequate to distinguish very tight stenosis from occlusion, although it may be useful as a screening test in the outpatient department. MRI angiography is fast becoming an important screening test, and CT with new reconstructive techniques such as "spiral" CT may also be used effectively.

The management of carotid atherosclerosis is best considered using a combination of clinical manifestations and angiographic pattern. Guidelines for treatment are presented in Table 12.1. It should be emphasized that there is still controversy about such issues as the appropriate management of asymptomatic bruit. A recent cooperative study has strongly confirmed the importance of carotid endarterectomy for symptomatic tight stenosis or moderate stenosis of greater than 65%.

Acute carotid occlusion is often asymptomatic; when it produces symptoms these usually reflect emboli from the top of the occlusion. Angicoagulation for 1 to 6 weeks is the treatment of choice for acute carotid occlusion to prevent these emboli. Occurrence of TIAs or progressive stroke above the occluded carotid is considered by many surgeons an indication for superficial temporal to middle cerebral bypass, but current evidence indicates that this procedure does not change the natural history of the disease.

Table 12.1. A Paradigm for Carotid Disease Management

Clinical Syndrome	CT or MRI	Angiography	Treatment
Asymptomatic bruit	no low absorption	ulcer	antiplatelet agents
	no low absorption	< 65% stenosis	observation
	no low absorption	> 65% stenosis	endarterectomy
Transient monocular blindness	+/− low absorption	complex ulcer	endarterectomy
or transient hemisphere	+/− low absorption	< 65% stenosis	anticoagulation
attack	+/− low absorption	> 65% stenosis	endarterectomy
Stroke	low absorption	ulcer	endarterectomy
	low absorption	< 65% stenosis	anticoagulation
	low absorption*	> 65% stenosis	endarterectomy

*Surgery is indicated only if the patient is not drowsy and does not have a major deficit

A tight carotid stenosis (less than 1 mm residual lumen) presents several management options. Recent evidence suggests that narrowing over 65% is best treated with endarterectomy, however. An ulcerated plaque is best treated with antiplatelet agents or anticoagulation unless the ulcer is very deep or symptoms have continued despite the use of these agents.

The major procedure used to treat carotid artery atherosclerosis is carotid endarterectomy, an operation in which the common, external, and internal carotid arteries are cross-clamped, opened, and cleaned of atherosclerotic plaque. Usually this procedure is done with electroencephalographic monitoring to detect ischemia during the period of clamping the artery, but some argue that this is not necessary. Surgeons also disagree about whether to use a shunt to maintain carotid flow during the removal of plaque. Proponents say it lessens ischemia; opponents argue that its insertion may increase emboli and that temporary occlusion is well tolerated. The surgery is relatively safe in experienced hands, with an overall morbidity of 5–10 percent and mortality of 1 to 2 percent. The major complications are postoperative or intraoperative cerebral emboli and myocardial infarction. Such angiographic characteristics as contralateral carotid occlusion, a high bifurcation, and tandem stenosis in the carotid siphon make the surgery riskier, as does poor medical condition.

Bypass grafting of external carotid to internal carotid is not presently used for treating ischemia because of lack of efficacy demonstrated in a cooperative study.

Atherosclerosis in the Vertebrobasilar System

Ischemic disease in the vertebrobasilar system usually means occlusion of the basilar artery or a small basilar branch. As in the anterior circulation, it is useful to look at specific disease syndromes here, beginning with the vertebral artery.

Two syndromes referable to the vertebral artery may be overrated as causes of symptoms. The first is subclavian steal, which is said to occur when flow to the arm is "stolen" from the vertebral artery because there is narrowing of the subclavian artery proximal to the vertebral takeoff. The result is vertebrobasilar ischemic symptoms; in fact, ischemic symptoms arise more often from a stenotic carotid or vertebral artery than from subclavian steal. Second, cervical osteophytes are sometimes said to compress the vertebral artery in the neck. This is very rare although the artery may be torn by cervical spine fractures or kinked by manipulation. Fibrous dysplasia can affect the cervical portion of the vertebral artery as well.

Unilateral vertebral occlusion often produces a lateral medullary syndrome from occlusion of the posterior inferior cerebellar artery; ipsilateral limb ataxia, dizziness and nystagmus, facial pain, crossed sensory and motor findings, ipsilateral Horner's syndrome, and dysphagia are characteristic. The occlusion may also result in a cerebellar infarct. If there is cerebellar infarction, hemipheric edema may act like a hemorrhage and cause preventable death from posterior fossa pressure. Emergency surgical resection of the infarcted hemisphere may be lifesaving. A CT scan may be sensitive enough and done low enough in the posterior fossa to demonstrate infarction, but MRI is a more useful test. It is important to recognize this syndrome clinically. Headache, drowsiness, vomiting, and resistance to neck movement are early signs that should raise the suspicion of a cerebellar infarction in a patient with a lateral medullary syndrome.

Atherosclerosis of both vertebral arteries produces a hypoperfusion syndrome with brain stem deficits increasing in the sitting position. Medical therapy is of little help for the hypoperfusion state that results; extracranial to intracranial bypass procedures may be lifesaving as these patients do very poorly with any medical regimen.

Basilar artery stenosis produces lacunes from small vessel occlusion as a result of atherosclerosis. Weakness, numbness, and transient dipolopia may be the only signs. With basilar thrombosis, however, there are bilateral arm and leg weakness and eye signs that may progress to death or a "locked-in" state. Maintaining perfusion is critical; heparin is often used to prevent the propagation of clot distally.

Embolic Strokes

Intracranial emboli may come from the heart wall or valves, from the carotid or vertebral artery, or from other sources. Eighty percent of strokes caused by emboli are maximal at onset, 12 percent are stepwise, and the remainder are gradual or fluctuating. Echocardiography should be carried out if emboli are suspected; it may reveal akinesis, clot, aneurysm, or valve disease. Holter monitoring may show transient arrhythmias. Carotid non-invasive studies should also be performed in all cases of anterior embolic stroke.

Some syndromes are characteristically embolic. In the anterior circulation, syndromes of middle cerebral artery occlusion are embolic. The other common embolus is at the top of the basilar artery. This can produce basilar or posterior cerebral symptoms. If the embolus remains in the basilar tip, there will be midbrain and thalamic infarction, with abnormalities of pupils, eye movements, and paresis or paralysis. If there is bilateral posterior cerebral artery occlusion, the patient will be cortically blind, with agitated confusion and memory loss from hippocampal and limbic system dysfunction. If there is a unilateral posterior cerebral occlusion, there will be a hemianopia; with strokes in the left hemisphere, the patient will have difficulty reading, on the right difficulty recognizing faces. The treatment of embolic disease is usually systemic anticoagulation.

Strokes from Systemic Hypotension

Strokes resulting from systemic hypotension occur in what are known as border-zone areas in the cerebral cortex. These are the areas of "watershed" cortical supply between the anterior and middle, and between the middle and posterior cerebral arteries. With strokes in the anterior-middle watershed, common findings are weakness "like a man in a barrel" with shoulder and thigh involved more than hands and feet because the area of least supply is high on the convexity where the shoulder and thigh areas are represented on the cortex. In the posterior-middle cerebral watershed, visual deficit and memory difficulty are important findings because of hypothalamic and optic radiation involvement.

Intracerebral Hemorrhage

Intracerebral hemorrhages occur into brain parenchyma; they are characterized by vomiting, headache, and neurological deficit. In 67 percent of cases the deficit develops gradually. The most common causes are hypertension, anticoagulation, or other bleeding diathesis, and arteriovenous malformations. Aneurysms at the periphery of arteries from sepsis or trauma may also hemorrhage. Amyloidosis, characterized by multiple hemorrhages in older patients, is a rare cause but one that is important to recognize because of the likelihood of recurrence.

The major diagnostic tool in suspected hemorrhage is CT scanning. A scan should be obtained immediately in any such patients with headache, vomiting, and a new neurological deficit. Angiography to evaluate an occult AVM is not usually helpful in putamenal or thalamic hemorrhages but should be considered in lobar hemorrhages if urgent evacuation is not necessary.

Different sites of hemorrhage have characteristic patterns that should be learned carefully. The most important are syndromes that indicate surgically evacuable hemorrhages. Cerebellar hemorrhages, which comprise 10 percent of all intracerebral hemorrhages, present with difficulty walking, headache, vomiting, dizziness, and gaze paresis (with the eyes looking to the side of the hemorrhage). Findings on examination include ataxia, small pupils, dysarthria, and oculomotor palsy. Emergency evacuation can be lifesaving. Lobar hemorrhages, comprising about 20 percent of all cerebral hemorrhages, should be evacuated if they result in drowsiness or significant midline shift on CT. Especially in the temporal region they may be treacherous. Angiography should be done before surgery if the patient is stable because AVMs and aneurysms are potential causes.

Caudate hemorrhages present with behavioral disturbances and can be removed if they produce mass effect. Right putamenal hemorrhages may also benefit from surgery. Putamenal hemorrhages are common, comprising about 50 percent of all intracerebral hemorrhages: they arise from perforating vessels arising from the internal carotid. These hemorrhages present with hemiplegia and eye deviation to the side of the lesion. On the left, the risk of further damage to the speech areas involved in the initial injury may be a reason to avoid surgery; on the right, however, surgery may be lifesaving with a large hemorrhage and may lead to a satisfactory long-term outcome. Extension into the ventricle is in itself not a contraindication to surgery, as patients can recover completely from intraventricular hemorrhage alone.

For several intracerebral hemorrhages, surgery has no benefit. Thalamic hemorrhages, characterized by sensory deficits more profound than their motor counterparts, and by convergent eyes with small poorly reactive pupils, cannot be evacuated by open operation except by transversing the internal capsule. They are best left alone. Pontine hemorrhages produce coma and quadriplegia with pinpoint pupils, absent horizontal gaze, and preserved vertical gaze. Lateral tegmental hemorrhages produce ipsilateral Horner's syndrome, ataxia, hemisensory loss, and abnormal eye movements without much weakness. These hemorrhages generally resolve.

Hemorrhages that are in evacuable areas and produce drowsiness or significant midline shift should be evacuated. If there is any question about their effect, an intraparenchymal pressure monitor will assess this accurately and may guide a decision to operate.

Subarachnoid Hemorrhage

From whatever cause, subarachnoid hemorrhage (SAH) produces headache, photophobia, neck stiffness, and acute obtundation. Intracranial aneurysms cause 57 percent of SAH, hypertension 15 percent, and AVMs or unknown cause 28 percent.

Cerebral Aneurysms

An intracranial aneurysm is an abnormal localized dilatation of an artery within the skull. If all arterial dilatations larger than 3 mm are included, the incidence in autopsy series is 4 percent of patients. Aneurysms may be congenital, atherosclerotic, mycotic, or traumatic. Congenital (berry) aneurysms arise at the bifurcations of major intracranial vessels, especially the internal carotid, posterior communicating, and middle cerebral arteries. They are accompanied by thinning of the internal elastic lamina of the artery wall. Atherosclerotic (fusiform) aneurysms involve diffuse widening of a major cerebral vessel and are associated with widespread atherosclerotic disease. The basilar artery is most commonly affected. Mycotic aneurysms, which account for fewer than 5 percent of all intracranial aneurysms, are associated with septicemia and subacute bacterial endocarditis; infected emboli enlarge the vessel wall by destroying important structural components. Neoplastic aneurysms have a similar mechanism. Mycotic aneurysms are usually treated with antibiotics and observation; recently, however, there has been a tendency to clip them if they are accessible or certainly if they enlarge. Traumatic aneurysms occur with gunshot or knife wounds or trauma. They should be explored and resected or otherwise repaired as soon as they are identified.

Fifty percent of patients with ruptured aneurysms present with the subarachnoid hemorrhage syndrome of headache, photophobia, neck stiffness, and loss of consciousness. Subdural hematomas and intracerebral hemorrhage may also be the earliest sign; occasionally a cranial nerve palsy, especially of the third nerve, is the first sign of a large internal carotid artery aneurysm.

A CT scan is the best initial diagnostic step; it often shows cisternal blood and occasionally the aneurysm itself. Lumbar puncture is not a necessary step for the diagnosis if the CT scan indicates subarachnoid blood. Furthermore, lumbar puncture may cause recurrent rupture. The CSF is usually bloody but may take 4 hours after hemorrhage to become so. After 24 hours, the CSF becomes xanthochromic. Angiography is the definitive study and should be done quickly so that early surgery can be performed when appropriate. MRI angiography is a good initial screen if available.

The first month after ruptured intracranial aneurysm is dangerous, with a mortality rate of 50 percent. The major problems are rebleeding, vasospasm, and hydrocephalus. Rebleeding occurs in up to 23 percent of patients in the first 4 weeks. Vasospasm refers both to angiographic arterial narrowing and to ischemic focal complications after SAH. Angiographic narrowing occurred in 74 percent of patients in one series; it usually involves the region occupied by blood clot and is related to clot around the blood vessel concerned. Ischemic complications can vary from transient vasoconstriction to coma and death. Hydrocephalus of mild degree is common and requires shunting in about 20 percent of cases. Clinical grading is a helpful guide to management. Table 12.2 summarizes one classification.

Early surgery is preferable, since it allows more effective treatment of vasospasm (induced hypertension, hemodilution, hypervolemia, nimodipine) and reduces the risk of rebleeding, which is high-

Table 12.2. Hunt-Hess Classification of Patients with SAH

Grade I	asymptomatic or minimal headache with nuchal rigidity
Grade Ia	fixed neurologic deficit
Grade II	moderate to severe headache, nuchal rigidity, no neurological deficit except cranial nerve palsy
Grade III	drowsiness, confusion, or new mild focal deficit
Grade IV	stupor, moderate to severe hemiparesis, early decerebrate rigidity, or vegetative disturbance
Grade V	deep coma, decerebrate rigidity, morbid appearance

est in the first 24–48 hours after a subarachnoid hemorrhage. The probability of rebleeding within the first 24 hours is approximately 4 percent, dropping to 1.5 percent per day for a total risk of 20 percent during the initial 14 days after hemorrhage. In the International Cooperative Study on the Timing of Aneurysm Surgery, outcome for early (1–3 days post-bleed) and late (11–14 days) surgery did not differ. This indicates that early surgery can be done safely.

The surgical procedure of choice for cerebral aneurysms is direct aneurysm clipping using microsurgical technique. Careful anesthetic technique with controlled ventilation is needed including meticulous avoidance of hypertension. The aneurysm is dissected at its junction with the parent artery and important neighboring branches are identified. The neck is clipped. If the neck cannot be clipped, carotid ligation is an alternative, especially in aneurysms over 3 cm in diameter. This may be associated with ischemic and embolic complications and should be done only by surgeons experienced in its use.

Interventional radiology is a potential alternative to surgery for some aneurysms, especially those of the posterior circulation.

Results and Complications

Vasospasm, hydrocephalus, and clip slippage are possible problems. In expert hands, however, operative mortality for aneurysm clipping in patients in good condition is about 2 percent; even for basilar aneurysms it is 8 percent in experienced hands.

Intracranial Arteriovenous Malformations

Definition

Arteriovenous malformations are abnormal collections of blood vessels. True arteriovenous malformations have both anomalous arterial structures, often with loss of normal elastic and muscle fibers, and dilated venous channels. They can be distinguished pathologically from cavernous angiomas, which have large sinusoidal spaces and intervening parenchyma; venous malformations, which lack arterial structures and are therefore low flow channels; and capillary telangiectases, which have very small channels. Venous malformations and capillary telangiectases are not operative lesions since they are not likely to be clinically significant. Neural parenchyma between small channels distinguishes telangiectases from cavernous angiomas.

Clinical Presentation

There are three typical presentations: 1) subarachnoid hemorrhage or intracerebral hemorrhage (in 50% of patients); 2) seizure, about as common; and 3) a slowly progressive neurological deficit (rare). Many patients note headache in retrospect, but it is not characteristic. A minority of patients have an intracranial bruit.

Diagnostic Tests

CT scanning may demonstrate the malformation or lead to a suspicion of one due to the pattern of intracerebral hemorrhage. Angiography of all vessels is the diagnostic procedure of choice; large feeding arteries, a malformed vascular bed, and enlarged drainage veins characterize the lesion. A vascular glioma may mimic an AVM but has more mass effect on CT.

Surgery

Surgery is not emergent unless there is a life-threatening hematoma. It is undertaken with preoperative corticosteroids, angiography, and wide cranial exposure. Feeding vessels are ligated first and great care must be taken to remove the entire malformation, since residual fragments will usually cause postoperative hemorrhage.

Several adjuncts to surgery have been proposed including embolization with fragments of gelfoam or plastic, or filling with methacrylate. These techniques are still evolving. The best treatment remains complete surgical extirpation. For smaller AVMs (2 cm or less) in surgically inaccessible locations, radiosurgery offers an effective alternative that appears to work by inducing endothelial hyperplasia and thrombosis of the lesion over several years.

The decision to operate on an AVM is a difficult one that must take into account the patient's age and deficits (both current and potential), the history, and the surgeon's experience. It is estimated that the rate of spontaneous hemorrhage in previously unruptured

AVMs is 2–3 percent per year and that mortality for such hemorrhages is 10 percent. These figures must be weighed against the risk of surgery.

Two other procedures have advocates in AVM management: 1) radiosurgery, either with linear accelerator or gamma knife; and 2) angiographically-guided embolization. These are available only in specialized centers but appear to be effective alternatives when appropriate.

Vascular Diseases of the Spinal Cord

Vascular diseases do not occur as frequently in the spinal cord as they do in the brain. Aneurysms are virtually never found in spinal arteries. Several recent advances have been made in understanding spinal arteriovenous malformations (AVMs). These advances have significantly altered the management of most patients with spinal AVMs and have lead to new treatments and better outcomes. Patients with spinal AVMs can present with acute spinal cord dysfunction as a result of hemorrhage or with chronic progression of myelopathy in a subacute manner. There are three main types of vascular malformations of the spine: dural arteriovenous fistula, in which the nidus of the AV fistula is embedded in the dural covering of the nerve root and the adjacent spinal dura; intradural vascular malformations, in which the nidus is either located within the tissue of the spinal cord or embedded in the pia; and cavernous angiomas. Intradural vascular malformations can be further classified as juvenile and glomus AVMs.

Magnetic resonance imaging has now replaced myelography as the first diagnostic procedure in patients with spinal AVMs. MR imaging can show serpentine areas of low signal intensity in the subarachnoid space reflecting blood flowing in the dilated vessels. However, the MRI can also be normal or reveal nonspecific abnormal signal in patients with a dural AV fistula. This type of spinal AVM is not only the most common, but it is the most amenable to treatment. Patients with a dural AV fistula can remain undiagnosed if investigation of myelopathy or radiculopathy is terminated after an MRI as the only diagnostic test.

In contrast to MRI, myelograms are universally abnormal and demonstrate the presence of a lesion in patients with all types of spinal vascular malformations except cavernous angiomas. Therefore, there is no need to search for a spinal AVM with arteriography in patients with a negative myelogram. However, if an MRI or myelogram points to the diagnosis of a spinal AVM, spinal arteriography should then be performed to better delineate the anatomy of the malformation.

The goal of treatment in patients with a dural AV fistula is to eliminate the venous congestion. Previously, it was not realized that the nidus of such AV fistulas is in the dura. Therefore, it was common to attempt to strip the engorged coronal venous plexus from the surface of the spinal cord. This procedure required an extensive laminectomy and is now deemed an unnecessary operation. The operation of choice now is to surgically interrupt the vessel that carries blood from the dural fistula to the coronal venous plexus. This can be accomplished by a simple hemilaminectomy. After the proximal nerve root ganglion has been exposed, the dura is opened and the site of intradural penetration of the vein draining the AV fistula is identified. The vessel is almost always adjacent to the site of dural penetration of the nerve root. The intradural draining vessel is then coagulated with bipolar cautery. This is probably sufficient therapy in most patients; it eliminates venous congestion of the cord without endangering the cord vascularity or the function of the nerve root at the involved level. The treatment of intradural spinal AVMs is more difficult and can be aided by embolization.

Other spinal disorders related to blood vessels include subdural and epidural hematomas, both of which can occur spontaneously, especially in patients on anticoagulants. The CT is **not** helpful in their diagnosis. Emergency myelography or MRI should be ordered if there is a history of back pain and neurological deterioration. This should be followed by emergency decompression.

Suggestions for Further Reading

The CASANOVA Study Group. Carotid surgery versus medical therapy in asymptomatic carotid stenosis. *Stroke* 22:1229–1235, 1991.

Ojemann RG, Heros RC, and Crowell R. *Surgical Management of Cerebrovascular Disease.* Second ed. Baltimore: Williams & Wilkins, 1988.

Samson DS and Batjer HH. *Intracranial Aneurysm Surgery: Techniques.* Mount Kisco, New York: Futura, 1990.

Toole JF. *Cerebrovascular Disorders*. Fourth ed. New York: Raven Press, 1990.

Wilkins RH. Natural history of arteriovenous malformations of the brain. In Barrow DL, *Intracranial Vascular Malformations*. Chicago: American Association of Neurological Surgeons, 1990, pp. 31–44.

13

Infections of the Brain and Spine

Cerebral Infections

Infections can occur in every region of the brain and its covering; each type has different implications for neurosurgical care.

Bone Infections

Bone infections usually occur after a craniotomy or head injury. A skull X-ray will show a moth-eaten appearance of the bone. Unfortunately, this is not too different from the appearance of a normal bone flap that has a limited blood supply so that it is difficult on X-ray alone to make this differential diagnosis. An indium-labeled white blood cell scan may be helpful in this situation. Usually patients with osteomyelitis have tenderness or puffiness over the affected bone and may have a draining sinus tract as well; they often have fever. The treatment for osteomyelitis is antibiotics, but if the bone is disconnected from other pieces of bone it must be removed and a bone flap that is infected needs to be removed. Cranioplasty can be done 6 months or more after the infection has cleared.

Epidural Abscess

An epidural abscess is important to recognize early although it is not as imminently life-threatening as subdural empyema. It is usually associated with a sinus infection and shows up as a high- or low-signal abnormality epidurally on MRI. Patients are moderately sick with fever and headaches and may have some tenderness over the affected scalp region.

Subdural Empyema

Subdural empyema is a life-threatening condition that must be recognized and treated early. It is characterized by seizures, fever, and a feeling of extreme malaise. These may occur at a time when the CT scan or MRI is essentially unremarkable at first glance. There is usually, however, a low-signal rim over the cortex of the brain. Subdural empyema must be suspected when a patient is sick with fever, headache, and stiff neck. The presence of seizures as well makes the index of suspicion much higher. Subdural empyema must be treated by evacuation and prolonged antibiotics with irrigation of the cavity. *Staphylococcus* or *streptococcus* are the usual bacteria and should be treated accordingly.

Intracerebral Abscess

Intracerebral abscess, also a life-threatening condition, is treacherous because it tends not to present with infective signs; very often the symptoms are those of a mass and the CT appearance is simply one of an intracerebral mass with a low-density center. About one-third of abscesses result from sinusitis of some type. Frontal or ethmoid sinuses tend to be associated with frontal abscesses and mastoid air cells; mastoiditis tends to be associated with temporal lobe or cerebellar abscesses. About one-third of abscesses are from direct trauma, usually depressed open skull fracture or retained intracranial foreign bodies. About 15 percent of abscesses are from heart disease or systemic infection. Oral infections also can produce intracerebral abscesses, usually with anaerobic organisms. About 10 percent of abscesses are from prior neurosurgery, including shunts or craniotomy; it is crucial to have a high index of suspicion after any neurosurgical operation.

The first treatment for an intracerebral abscess is either aspiration or excision, depending on its location. Although excision has been favored in the past, the better availability of stereotactic techniques and the increasing ability to treat abscesses with antibiotics have advanced the view that minimal neurosurgical intervention may be preferable to full excision. A culture should be obtained for aerobic and anaerobic organisms. A rough guide to antibiotics is that wound infection abscesses are usually *staphylococcus aureus* or *streptococcus* infections, although anaerobic *streptococcus* may be involved. Abscesses with an oral source are often fusibacterium or bacteroides infections. Abscesses associated with congenital heart disease may represent any sort of infection, but are often streptococcus, staphylococcus, or anaerobic. Abscesses from sinusitis often harbor gram negative organisms; those from the lung may be Klebsiella or other difficult organisms.

The CT scan is a useful tool in following a brain abscess, although it may lag behind resolution of the abscess by several weeks. In general 8–10 weeks of antibiotics are required to be certain the abscess has been completely treated.

AIDS in the Brain

The infections that are associated with AIDS are of increasing importance in neurosurgery. The occurrence of multiple enhancing nodules on MRI or CT in a young or middle-aged patient should make one suspicious of this problem even in patients without known HIV infection. The most common brain infection in a patient who has known AIDS is toxoplasmosis. Empirical treatment for this disorder with sulfaxozasole is often indicated as the first step. If this does not result in some diminution of lesions within 2 months, stereotactic biopsy is usually considered. Low-density areas in a patient with AIDS may be toxoplasmosis, lymphoma, or AIDS infection itself.

Herpes Encephalitis

Herpes simplex encephalitis tends to localize in the temporal and orbitofrontal lobes and often results in hemorrhagic necrosis. The most common findings are fever, personality change, and seizures. CT scan can be helpful in diagnosis, showing evidence of a hemorrhagic lesion. Early diagnosis is important because acyclovir is an effective treatment; it must be started early to prevent long-term sequelae.

Creutzfeld-Jakob Disease

This disease is important to recognize because of its potential for infecting the neurosurgeon. It is caused by a slow virus that gradually destroys the brain parenchyma in characteristic vacuolar degeneration. Atrophy on CT or MRI is the imaging picture, and dementia and myoclonus are characteristic clinical patterns. Instruments that have been used for biopsy must be processed by special techniques.

Spine Infections

Osteomyelitis

Osteomyelitis of a vertebral body is characterized by pain, spasms, and sometimes by systemic symptoms of fever or chills. It most often follows sepsis; the most common organism is *staphylococcus aureus*. CT or MRI will show erosion of the bone. Osteomyelitis can be diagnosed by bone biopsy. Treatment consists of a 6-week course of appropriate intravenous antibiotics. Tuberculous osteomyelitis or Pott's disease is particularly problematic; plain X-rays show a moth-eaten appearance of bone that often involves the disc space. A paraspinous mass may also be visible on radiographic studies.

Disc Space Infection

Disc space infections are most common in the lumbar spine; they can occur following disc removal or lumbar puncture. They may also occur spontaneously. Their hallmark is severe low back pain and spasm. The temperature and peripheral white count are only slightly elevated but the erythrocyte sedimentation rate is always elevated. A physical exam may reveal only local tenderness and muscle spasm. Bacterial cultures, which may be obtained by disc space biopsy, are positive in only half the cases. If bacteria are found, the most commonly cultured organism is a *Staphylococcus* species. Two to six weeks after symptoms begin, X-rays will show destruction of adjacent vertebral bodies. Ultimately, there is bony fusion of the two adjacent vertebrae. Initial treatment includes bed rest, immobilization, and analgesic medications. Intravenous antibiotics are used by most physicians as well.

Spinal Epidural and Subdural Abscesses

These rare problems have an importance far beyond their incidence. They occur most often after septicemia or osteomyelitis. Patients with an epidural abscess usually have a history of back pain, fever, leukocytosis, and spinal tenderness. Once neurological changes begin, the usual course is rapid deterioration to paralysis. This is most often irreversible, so a premium must be placed on early recognition. Severe back pain with fever and tenderness must be considered signs of an epidural abscess until myelography or MRI excludes this entirely. MRI shows a high-signal epidural mass. Myelography may determine the diagnosis by demonstrating purulence at lumbar puncture. The myelogram will show an epidural compressive lesion that is not as impressive as the neurological deficit. It is advisable to inject dye from above as well as below if a lesion is found in order to define its length. Treatment is by wide laminectomy and drainage, followed by bed rest and 6 weeks of antibiotics. Usually the wound can be closed primarily.

A spinal subdural abscess is even more treacherous than an epidural abscess and fortunately even rarer. It presents with pain and neurological deficit but little back tenderness. Diagnosis is by MR. Treatment is the same as for epidural abscess.

Suggestions for Further Reading

Brown WJ and Voge M. *Neuropathology of Parasitic Infections.* New York: Oxford University Press, 1982.

Levy RM and Rosenblum ML. Neurosurgical aspects of human immunodeficiency virus (HIV-1) infection. In Wilkins RH and Rengachary SS, *Neurosurgery Update II.* New York: McGraw-Hill, 1991, pp. 257–268.

Johnson RT. *Viral Infections of the Nervous System.* New York: Raven Press, 1982.

Schlossberg D. *Infections of the Nervous System.* New York: Springer-Verlag, 1990.

14

Adult Cerebrospinal
Fluid Abnormalities

Adult Hydrocephalus

Adult hydrocephalus represents a spectrum of disorders ranging from the asymptomatic patient with large ventricles on CT to a very ill patient in coma after subarachnoid hemorrhage. It is caused by an obstruction to CSF flow or outflow that may be acute or chronic. The most common acute causes are subarachnoid hemorrhage, trauma, and intracranial surgery; among others are cerebellar hemorrhage and tumors obstructing the ventricular system. Chronic causes include intracranial infections and idiopathic normal pressure hydrocephalus. Virtually all adult hydrocephalus is obstructive; that is, it involves a block to CSF passage within the brain.

A classification of hydrocephalus that is relevant to lumbar punctures and lumboperitoneal shunting is the distinction between communicating and noncommunicating hydrocephalus. In communicating hydrocephalus, the ventricular system is in continuity with the subarachnoid space; in noncommunicating hydrocephalus, there is an obstruction at some point in the pathway. Table 14.1 lists the causes of noncommunicating hydrocephalus. Lesions associated with communicating hydrocephalus are presented in Table 14.2.

Four clinical syndromes can be distinguished:

1. *Acute hydrocephalus* in which nausea, vomiting, headache, and progressive obtundation may progress over hours.
2. *Chronic high pressure hydrocephalus* in which headaches, papilledema, vomiting, behavioral disturbances, and visual loss

Table 14.1. Some Causes of Noncommunicating Hydrocephalus

A. Congenital lesions
   1. Aqueductal anomalies (gliosis, narrowing, forking, septum)
   2. Dandy-Walker cyst (atresia of the foramina of Luschka and Magendie)
   3. Posterior fossa tumors or cysts
   4. Arteriovenous malformations or other masses in brain stem or cerebellum

B. Acquired lesions
   1. Aqueductal stenosis
   2. Vascular malformations
   3. Tumors of the ventricles or posterior fossa

are present for weeks or months, and examination may reveal gait disturbance and failure of upgaze.

3. *Normal-pressure hydrocephalus (NPH),* in which the ventricles are large, there is minimal cortical atrophy and CSF pressure is normal. In adults, this condition is manifested by slowing of thought and action, dementia, urinary incontinence, and gait disturbance. In some cases gait disturbance may be the only sign. The condition characteristically follows subarachnoid hemorrhage, head trauma, or meningeal infections.

4. *Arrested hydrocephalus,* in which large ventricles and normal lumbar puncture pressure are not associated with any neurological findings, or only with mild diminution of intellectual capacities.

Table 14.2. Lesions Associated with Communicating Hydrocephalus

A. Congenital processes
   1. Arnold-Chiari malformation
   2. Encephalocele
   3. Inflammations of the meninges
   4. Lissencephaly (agyria)
   5. Congenital absence of arachnoid granulations

B. Acquired lesions
   1. Subarachnoid or ventricular hemorrhage
   2. Infections
   3. Trauma
   4. Ventricular or convexity masses
   5. Platybasia

C. Idiopathic

Diagnosis

A CT scan is the logical screening procedure in the diagnosis of adult hydrocephalus. An unenhanced scan will show the ventricular contour, and intravenous contrast injection may show a tumor or other lesion responsible for hydrocephalus. Ventriculography, pneumoencephalography, and angiography have no place in diagnosing and following hydrocephalus today. MRI provides better information than CT; ventricular volumes can be measured, the aqueduct can be visualized, and with new software programs CSF pulsatility and flow can be assessed, but this is expensive for routine management.

After a known event such as subarachnoid hemorrhage, diagnosing hydrocephalus is easy and shunting is virtually always indicated in the treatment of ventricular enlargement. The major diagnostic difficulty occurs in apparent normal-pressure hydrocephalus of unknown cause; here the distinction from Alzheimer's disease is not easy. The major distinguishing factor is the clinical predominance of gait disturbance in NPH, which also seems to correlate best with a good shunt response.

Radionuclide cisternography, usually done with indium DPTA, may help evaluate CSF dynamics; however, it has been of limited usefulness in hydrocephalus because a mixed pattern is the most common finding. Normally, intrathecal tracer does not enter the ventricles and ascends over the convexity in 12–24 hours. Retrograde filling of the ventricles, ("ventricular stasis"), and delayed or absent filling of the convexity subarachnoid spaces ("lack of convexity ascent") are typical of normal-pressure hydrocephalus. A mixed pattern shows only brief ventricular filling or some convexity ascent and is not helpful in diagnosing CSF obstruction.

Treatment

For hydrocephalus with elevated pressure, shunting is very successful at resolving symptoms and signs due to pressure. In normal-pressure hydrocephalus, about 60 percent of patients with the typical presentation will improve. Contraindications to shunting include scalp infection, ventriculitis, and sepsis.

For ventricular shunting, the ventricle may be entered from a posterior burr hole 6 cm above the inion and 3 cm to the right of midline. Alternatively, the catheter can be frontally placed 11 cm behind the glabella, 3 cm to the right of midline. Valve systems vary in design and pressure; specifications are available on manufacturers' inserts. In a ventriculoatrial shunt, tubing is inserted in the jugular vein and threaded to the junction of the superior vena cava and atrium. In the ventriculoperitoneal shunt it is placed in the peritoneal cavity. Meticulous sterile technique must be observed.

CSF Fistulas

CSF fistulas are a challenge to the neurosurgeon because they may be difficult both to localize and to repair. They may occur spontaneously, postoperatively, or after trauma. Spontaneous fistulae are the rarest; they may result from local erosion of bone and dura by a tumor or an aneurysm, diffusely increased intracranial pressure with leakage from the cribriform plate, congenital weakness of the cribriform plate, an empty sella, or an encephalocele. Postoperative fistulas may result from intracranial, spinal, or trans-sphenoidal pituitary surgery. Fistulae after trauma occur in 2 to 3 percent of all patients with head injuries. In 85 percent rhinorrhea ceases spontaneously within a week. Otorrhea virtually always ceases spontaneously. The cribriform plate is the most common site of CSF leakage in trauma, followed by frontal, ethmoid, and sphenoid fractures. Paradoxical rhinorrhea from a petrous fracture dripping via the eustachian tubes to the nose occasionally occurs.

Loss of smell and an air fluid level behind the tympanic membrane are suggestive of a CSF fistula. Free-flowing, watery, clear fluid from the nose is diagnostic if the chloride level is higher than it is in blood.

CSF leak may also be occult. One bout of meningitis after surgery or trauma, or more than one episode of meningitis in an adult without apparent cause, should suggest a hidden CSF leak. Investigation should include skull films, which may show intracranial air or a fracture; thin-section CT through the skull base both transaxially and coronally; and a RISA Indium or fluorescein CSF study with dye inserted via lumbar puncture and nasally placed sinus pledgets to detect the leak.

In treating CSF fistulas, the following principles may be applied (see Tables 14.3 and 14.4):

1. There is no good evidence that prophylactic antibiotics help. If they are used, oxacillin or nafcillin, effective against *strepto-*

Table 14.3. Management of Spontaneous CSF Leak (after Spetzler)

Associated Problem	High CSF Pressure	Normal CSF Pressure
With a space occupying lesion	remove mass	remove mass and repair dura
Hydrocephalus	shunt	shunt if clinically indicated
Congenital anomalies	repair +/− shunt	repair anomaly
Empty sella	pack sella	pack sella

coccus and *staphylococcus,* the two most common virulent organisms, should be chosen rather than a broad-spectrum drug because of the problem of drug-resistant infections.

2. Repair of facial trauma should be prompt to avoid a potential fistula.
3. Increased CSF pressure should be reduced if there is an accompanying CSF leak. Repeat lumbar punctures, lumbar drainage, or CSF shunting may be necessary in hydrocephalus; intracranial masses should be removed.
4. It may be helpful to lower normal CSF pressure to subnormal levels by a lumbar drain if there is a fistula; pneumocephalus is a danger, however, from air entering the head through the site of the leak.
5. Rough guidelines for surgical repair are as follows. In general, the CSF pressure should be normalized before direct repair is

Table 14.4. Management of Posttraumatic or Postsurgical CSF Leak

Cause of Leak	High CSF Pressure	Normal CSF Pressure
Traumatic		
immediate	normalize pressure	wait 10 days
delayed	shunt, then repair	repair
Surgical		
intracranial	shunt, then repair	repair
Trans-sphenoidal		
immediate	normalize pressure	wait 4 days, then repair
delayed	normalize pressure	repair
Lumbar puncture		blood patch

considered. Posttraumatic CSF leaks that do not stop in 10 days should be repaired. Even if they stop spontaneously, there is a potential danger of meningitis as brain may protrude into the bony defect. A postoperative CSF leak from trans-sphenoidal surgery may be given 4 to 7 days to resolve before being repaired by repacking the sella; lumbar drainage may facilitate its stoppage. A postoperative leak after cranial surgery will probably require repair if it lasts longer than 10 days. If it occurs through the incision, oversewing should be tried first.

6. Trans-sphenoidal or trans-ethmoidal surgery may be the approach of choice if the leak is localized to the sphenoid or ethmoid sinuses. Anosmia and often the complications of bifrontal craniotomy may be avoided by these routes.

7. If an intracranial procedure is required, it should be tailored to suit the problem. To obliterate a known leak, a skin and bone flap suited to it should be used. If the leak is large, midline or unknown, a bifrontal flap is necessary and it may also allow middle fossa exploration. Bone is repaired with bone wax, wire mesh, or methyl methacrylate under the tear; a pericranial, temporalis fascia, or fascia lata graft is placed over the defect and held to the dura with small stitches or glue. If no leak is identified, the sphenoid sinus can be obliterated by removing the tuberculum sella and packing it with fat or muscle. Tables 14.3 and 14.4 present management guidelines for leaks through bone or the incision.

Pseudotumor Cerebri

Pseudotumor cerebri is not clearly a CSF disorder, it is included in this chapter because it is a disorder of intracranial pressure. It is defined as increased intracranial pressure without a mass lesion or ventricular enlargement. Conditions associated with it are numerous (venous drainage obstruction, endocrine dysfunction, vitamin A excess or deficiency, anemia, drug reactions, steroid withdrawal) but its cause is unknown. Symptoms include headache, dizziness, nausea, tinnitus, and diplopia. Pseudotumor cerebri occurs most frequently in obese women aged 30–40. Its major danger is visual loss, which may occur in up to 40 percent of cases. Treatment with corticosteroids, acetazolamide, and glycerol has been tried with varying success. Serial lumbar punctures may help, but a lumboperitoneal shunt is usually corrective and should be carried out if visual loss is occurring.

Arachnoid Cysts

These cysts develop within the arachnoid membrane and may or may not communicate with cerebrospinal fluid. They are benign compressive lesions whose manifestations depend on their location. The Sylvian fissure is the most common site; headaches and rarely seizures occur. A cyst here may also result in a subdural hematoma. A CT scan is usually diagnostic, showing a smooth-walled structure of CSF density with no enhancement in the wall; however, it may be difficult to distinguish these from epidermoid cysts. Cerebral convexity cysts may produce seizures, headache, papilledema, and contralateral hemiparesis. Suprasellar arachnoid cysts may erode the sella and cause obstructive hydrocephalus, visual field cuts, and visual impairments. Here the CT may not show the lesion; metrizamide cisternography may be necessary. Cysts of the optic nerve sheath may lead to diminished visual acuity and papilledema. Suprapineal recess cysts produce hydrocephalus and Parinaud's syndrome (paralysis of upward gaze due to midbrain tectal compression). Cerebellopontine angle cysts cause hearing loss, posterior fossa compressive signs, and occasionally facial pain as well. Midline cerebellar cysts produce increased intracranial pressure and truncal ataxia.

Extradural spinal arachnoid cysts tend to occur in the midthoracic region, leading to kyphosis, slowly progressive paraparesis, and poorly defined sensory changes less severe than the motor effects. Spine X-rays may show bony erosion; myelography or MRI shows an extradural mass. Spinal arachnoid cysts may also develop along lumbar and sacral nerve roots.

The treatment of arachnoid cysts consists of widely opening the cyst wall and connecting it to an adjacent CSF space. Another option is to shunt the cyst.

Suggestions for Further Reading

Black P McL. Hydrocephalus in adults. In Youmans JR (ed). *Neurological Surgery*. Fourth ed. New York: Saunders, 1994.
Black P McL, Ojemann RG, and Tzouras A. CSF shunts for dementia, in-

continence, and gait disturbance. *Clin. Neurosurg.* 32:632–651, 1985.

Johnston I, Hawke S, Halmagyi M, and Teo C. The pseudotumor syndrome: Disorders of cerebrospinal fluid circulation causing intracranial hypertension without ventriculomegaly. *Arch. Neurol.* 48:740–747, 1991.

Post EM. Shunt systems. In Wilkins RH and Rengachary SS, *Neurosurgery Update II.* New York: McGraw-Hill, 1991, pp. 300–308.

Scott RM. *Hydrocephalus.* Baltimore: Williams and Wilkins, 1990.

Spetzler RF and Zabramski JM. Cerebrospinal fluid fistulae: their management and repair. In Youmans JR (ed). *Neurological Surgery.* Third Ed. Philadelphia: Saunders, 1990, 2269–2289.

15

Degenerative Diseases of the Spine

Intervertebral Disc Disease

Intervertebral disc disease is a common cause of neurological disability. It generally affects those segments of the spinal column that are most vulnerable to physical forces; the neck and lower back. In the neck, C5, C6, and C7 are most often involved; L4, L5, and S1 are the levels most commonly affected in the lower back. The thoracic spine, buttressed by the ribs, rarely suffers disc herniation, but it must be recognized and treated correctly when it occurs.

Cervical Disc Disease

The biochemical and physiological changes that accompany cervical disc disease are poorly understood. In young patients, cervical disc disease usually presents as an "acute disc" resulting in a radiculopathy characterized by neck and arm pain. The fissuring of the firm annulus fibrosis that surrounds the more compressible nucleus pulposis may allow lateral extrusion of a fragment of soft ruptured disk with no particular antecedent. A variant of the acute form is central rather than lateral herniation and it can result in a myelopathy as well as radiculopathy. In older patients, cervical disc disease generally has a more chronic course, with gradual degeneration of the disc and surrounding bones and recurrent episodes of arm or neck pain. This form of chronic disc disease are known as cervical spondylosis. The degenerative process of cervical spondylosis includes the thinning and bulging of discs themselves as well as the development of bony ridges or "osteophytes" between vertebral bodies, especially at the uncinate processes which lie beside the neural formaniae. Hypertrophy of the so-called apophyseal or facet joints, which provide the posterolateral stabilizing columns for the cervical spine, may further narrow the neural foramina. The usual levels affected by either acute or chronic cervical disc disease are C5–6, C6–7, and C7–T1.

The effects of acute and chronic cervical disc disease are similar: nerve root compression (radiculopathy) with lateral herniation of disc material, or spinal cord compression (myelopathy) by posterior extrusion of disc or by gradual encroachment of bony osteophytes upon the spinal canal. The major distinguishing clinical features between acute and chronic disc disease are the mode of onset (rapid in the first, more gradual in the second) and severity of pain (excruciating in the first, waxing and waning in the second).

The characteristic clinical features of cervical root compression are pain, paresthesias, and weakness. Neck pain with tenderness worse on motion is often accompanied by headache. Pain may radiate into the shoulder, chest, arm, or hand. There may also be numbness or tingling in the arm, forearm, or hand. Because the roots exit directly opposite the disc space, a C5–6 disc will compress the C6 nerve root, C6–7 the C7 root, and C7–T1 the C8 root. Weakness and paresthesias are more helpful than the symptom of pain radiation in establishing the level of involvement. C6 compression gives pain in the lateral arm and sometimes forearm with numbness and tingling in the thumb and index finger. The biceps on the affected side is weak and its reflex is depressed. C7 compression produces arm and forearm pain, weakness in the triceps, a diminished triceps reflex, and paresthesias into the middle finger. The latissimus dorsi is also weak on the side of the pain. C8 compression produces pain down the medial forearm ("medial" in terms of the anatomical position where the arm is supinated with palm open and forward). There is numbness in the ring and small finger, weak hand intrinsic muscles (lumbricals and interossei), and no reflex change. Less common syndromes occur with C5 compression, which produces pain from the side of the neck to shoulder tip, deltoid numbness, and weakness of shoulder extension; C4 compression, which leads to pain and numbness in the anterior chest and back of the neck; and C3 compression, which causes pain in the pinna of the ear.

Most acute and chronic pain episodes involving cervical radiculopathy and spondylosis will resolve with conservative, nonoperative treatment. Anti-inflammatory drugs such as ibuprofen and muscle relaxants are often useful. Many patients respond well to cervical traction, which can be done at home or in the physiotherapy department. For the best results, a chin strap is used with 7–8 pounds for half-hour intervals several times a day. Some patients find that traction worsens their pain; it should be discontinued under these circumstances. For particular pain sites, diathermy and ultrasound may help in the short term. Cervical isometric exercises (pushing against resistance for 5 seconds 15 times twice a day in front, back, and each side) may help in both acute and long-term care.

Cervical spine films are helpful in evaluating patients with neck pain. In acute herniation, there may be narrowing of a disc space with loss of normal curvature. In chronic disc disease there may be narrowing of the AP diameter of the canal (less than 11 mm is always pathological), foraminal encroachment, instability (subluxation over 3.5 mm is abnormal), and degeneration of the apophyseal joints. In patients older than 40, however, X-ray changes and clinical symptoms do not always correlate with each other.

Myelopathy, or spinal cord compression, is the other significant syndrome produced by cervical disc disease. Acutely, it can result from a large central herniation of disc material. There may or may not be neck pain followed by stiffening of gait, unsteadiness, hand clumsiness, and ultimately bladder dysfunction. MRI is the diagnostic method of choice. Urgent surgical resection should be carried out.

Chronic cervical myelopathy usually results from cervical spondylosis, bony thickening that appears to accompany chronic degenerative disease. Initially there is hand clumsiness and numbness followed by leg weakness and increased tone. There is a wide-based spastic gait. Reflexes are hyperactive below the spondylotic ridge. The jaw jerk is not hyperactive, a point that may distinguish spondylosis from amyotrophic lateral sclerosis, which may affect jaw jerk as well as other spinal reflexes. Abdominal reflexes are diminished and the toes may go either up or down. Bladder and bowel function are not usually impaired, which may be important in distinguishing cervical myelopathy from spinal cord tumor.

The best initial test for assessing cervical disc disease is MRI. With the right sequences it will provide both sagittal and transaxial views of the cervical canal, distinguishing disc disease from bony encroachment. Transaxially it permits assessment of nerve root compression by disc fragment or bone, but may not be fully sensitive to bony changes.

CT scanning with thin-section transaxial cuts is also useful in assessing clinical disc disease. It will establish whether there is soft disc disease or an osteophyte but will not provide information about the thecal sac. For this, contrast must be added to the subarachnoid space. Usually soluble contrast material is used and transaxial sections are made.

The electromyogram rarely helps localize the lesion to a specific nerve root. It may, however, reinforce the decision to do a myelogram or other imaging in a patient whose only symptom is pain, or help differentiate root compression from brachial plexus abnormalities. Discography is not generally considered useful, nor is lumbar puncture.

The indications for surgery for cervical disc disease and spondylosis vary from center to center, but several guidelines can be agreed upon. First, surgery is not generally helpful in patients with neck pain alone and no radiculopathy or myelopathy. Second, in evaluating a patient with an acutely painful neck, if the pain is severe and seems related to the rupture of an acute soft disc, early disc excision may be the best treatment. If bony encroachment is the cause, the surgical outcome is generally worse, and a longer trial of conservative therapy may be indicated. Third, both anterior and posterior approaches should be available to the neurosurgeon for the best overall management.

For a single lateral soft disc herniation, we prefer a posterior approach with laminotomy and disc fragment removal because the procedure has the least potential morbidity; however, anterior disc resection is done in many centers with equal success. For a central soft disc herniation or single-level hard bony spur osteophyte, most surgeons would agree that anterior discectomy and osteophyte removal are indicated. Fusion with autologous or donor bone may or may not be done. For multilevel osteophyte formation, which is the situation in most cases of spondylosis, there are widely disparate approaches. Some surgeons claim that anterior removal of osteophytes up to three levels will provide good decompression and stability; others prefer wide posterior decompression.

The surgical results vary depending on the etiology. Removal of a soft lateral disc herniation by a posterior approach is one of the most satisfying procedures in neurosurgery. Good results are often achievable by anterior disc removal as well, with at least partial resolution of myelopathy. For bony compression, the situation is less gratifying. Many patients experience relief of radicular pain, but neck pain may continue to plague them. Similarly, the relief of spondolytic myelopathy by decompressive laminectomy is often slight. Laminectomy may prevent further deterioration, but improvement in gait or sensation is rarely striking. Perhaps earlier surgery would prevent the long-term changes seen in patients with advanced bony change and cord disease. Clearly this important area needs further study.

Thoracic Disc Disease

Thoracic disc herniation is rare but important to recognize. The clinical presentation is chronic myelopathy, occasionally with radicular pain. Calcification of the disc space on plain spine films, a mass continuous with the disc space on CT or MRI, and a ventral defect opposite the disc space by myelogram are important clues to thoracic disc herniation. Laminectomy should *not* be done: it allows the cord to bulge backward and is associated with a significant incidence of postoperative paraplegia. The two acceptable approaches are posterolateral costotransversectomy or anterior discectomy by transthoracic approach. Experienced hands are necessary for either of these procedures.

Lumbar Disc Disease

Lumbar disc disease, in whatever form it presents, is best regarded as a chronic problem with acute exacerbations. The fundamental changes are degeneration of the intervertebral disc with weakening of the firm circumferential annulus and altered tension of the central nucleus pulposis. In young people, the usual presentation is rupture of a fragment of nucleus through the annulus, leading to acute compression of a nerve root; in patients over 40 there is likely to be a much more complex set of factors probably related to intervertebral disc degeneration. These changes include increased mobility between vertebrae, formation of ridges or osteophytes between vertebral bodies, overgrowth and degeneration of articular facets, and narrowing of the disc spaces. These symptoms may be complicated by congenital narrowing of the spinal canal.

There are four well-recognized clinical syndromes attributable to lumbar disc disease: recurrent low back pain, acute monoradiculopathy, cauda equina compression, and the "failed back." The most common is recurrent low back pain, often related to sitting or walking, usually associated with back spasm and limitation of motion. Without nerve root compression, this pain may nevertheless radiate into one or both legs as far as the knee. Treatment of this syndrome is conservative (see below). The second common syndrome is an acute monoradiculopathy. This presents as a pain radiating into the leg and foot, worse on coughing and sneezing. In the young patient it is usually a result of herniation of disc material against an exiting nerve root; in the older patient, it may represent acute root inflammation, swelling from rupture of a small disc fragment, or compression against bony overgrowth. This syndrome may be treated with bed rest or surgery. The third syndrome is an acute cauda equina syndrome, invoving sensory loss in the legs and bowel or bladder dysfunction. This is a neurosurgical emergency and requires urgent disc excision. The final syndrome is the so-called "failed back," with long term disabling pain, which often follows multiple surgical procedures and is very difficult to treat. Each of these will be discussed in more detail.

Little is understood about the biomechanics of the back that lead to chronic recurrent low back pain. In susceptible patients, it may be an incapacitating condition. Training in "back schools," including instruction in sitting, standing, lifting, occupational adjustment, and a back exercise program, seems the best therapy.

For acute lumbar disc rupture, the history is often diagnostic: sudden back and leg pain, worse on moving, sitting, coughing, or sneezing, and radiating beyond the knee. Examination demonstrates signs of root irritation, root compression, and root tension. Disc irritation is demonstrated by tenderness over the level affected and along the nerve as well as in muscles supplied by that root. Findings of root compression include loss of sensation, muscle strength, and reflex function. In L5–S1 disc rupture, the S1 root is usually compressed; there is numbness over the lateral foot and heel, diminished ankle jerk, weakness of foot plantar flexion, and atrophy of gastrocnemius and soleus muscles. In an L4–L5 disc rupture, the L5 root is compressed; sensation is diminished over the medial foot, with diminished ability to dorsiflex the foot and great toe and stand on the heel. Reflexes are usually preserved. In an L3–4 disc rupture, there is L4 root compression; sensory loss is in the posterolateral thigh and anteromedial leg, motor findings include weakness of knee extension and atrophy of thigh muscles, and the knee jerk is diminished. Atypical presentations are also seen.

Several tests of nerve tension have been devised. The most reliable is straight leg raising or Lasègue's test. If the leg on the affected side is elevated while the unaffected leg is kept straight, a ruptured disc will give pain radiating into the symptomatic leg and foot. A variant also described by Lasègue is to flex the knee and hip, then gradually extend the knee; again there will be leg and foot pain on the affected side. A third test, for the bowstring sign, reveals pain on knee extension on the affected side. Finger pressure on the popliteal space with the knee extended will also give pain. Crossed straight leg raising or Fajerstajn's sign, in which elevation of the asymptomatic leg causes pain in the painful leg and foot, is an important and reliable sign of disc rupture outside the annulus. Symptoms in this case are not likely to improve with rest.

These pain symptoms are important because they demonstrate acute mechanical irritation of the nerve roots. It is also critical to check the hip joint, abdomen, rectum, and pelvis to be certain that disc herniation is the cause of pain. Other lesions, far less common than disc disease but very important to diagnose, may produce radicular pain. These include intraspinal tumors such as conus ependymomas, nerve root neurofibromas or hemangiomas, epidural tumors that may be metastatic, and masses in the lumbosacral plexus. Atypical pain, especially pain worse on lying down, requires extensive investigation for these lesions including careful examination of the buttocks and CT of the entire pelvis.

The noninvasive evaluation of lumbar disc disease is now very satisfactory with MR and CT scanning. Both of these modalities demonstrate disc material and neural structures. MRI is the procedure of choice. Sagittal sections demonstrate disc rupture and its level; transaxial views permit evaluation of nerve roots and the dural sac. Disc material can be distinguished from synovial cysts and osteophytes and in some cases lateral disc herniations can be identified. The MRI should include the conus in its sagittal view to exclude pathology there. CT can lead to a false-positive interpretation if sections are not taken through the disc space, and for that reason a reconstruction format may be important to be certain of significant herniation. To be certain of the findings and to exclude intraspinal pathology elsewhere, many surgeons still do myelography for definitive diagnosis. This procedure has little morbidity if done with a water-soluble medium and a fine lumbar puncture needle. Persistence of nausea, vomiting, or headache after a myelogram suggest a CSF leak through the dural rent; this responds to an epidural blood patch if bed rest for a week is not sufficient. On the myelogram, a ruptured disc is seen as a smooth or irregular defect opposite the disc space, obliterating one or more nerve roots. The roots should be followed out carefully to find subtle impressions. The CT is better than myelography for indentifying very lateral ruptures. The region of the conus must be evaluated in all lumbar myelograms as well to exclude tumor.

The initial treatment of lumbar root irritation from disc rupture includes bed rest, analgesics or anti-inflammatory agents, and time. Bedrest should be on a firm mattress and should be as strict as is compatible with self-care. Analgesics should be as mild as possible, beginning with aspirin and moving on if necessary to propoxyphene, codeine, or demerol for the acute case. Strong narcotics such as demerol, morphine, or oxycodone should be prescribed very sparingly; their addiction potential in the treatment of chronic back pain is enormous. Anti-inflammatory agents such as ibuprofen, naprosyn, or butazolidine have a substantial role in acute management. The author's experience is that "antispasmodic" agents such as diazepam are useful primarily as tranquilizers, allowing prolonged bed rest.

This conservative program should be followed for at least 2 weeks and up to 6 weeks. If there is no improvement, further investigation and surgery should be considered. CT may be done while conservative treatment is being carried out to exclude a very large disc that may require resection. Other studies such as EMGs are not necessary but may help to establish radicular compression.

There is some disagreement about the indications for surgery with lumbar disc rupture and acute leg pain. Most surgeons agree that an acute neurological defect (e.g., foot drop) or intractable pain despite bed rest are best treated by surgery. There is disagreement about what constitutes a significant deficit and what pain is severe enough to warrant surgery. The decision to operate in lumbar disc disease requires careful surgical judgment.

Discectomy involves partial laminectomy and wide exposure of the disc and surrounding region. It allows removal of bone that may be acting as a compressive mass, careful exploration of the nerve root for any sequestered disc, and complete discectomy with minimal nerve root retraction. This operation can yield 85 percent satisfactory results when done for radicular pain. There may be a potential for greater instability associated with it than with microsurgical discectomy if the facet is disrupted; however, the recurrence rate of disc herniation is less. Several percutaneous discectomy techniques have been developed but are still evolving. Open discectomy remains the gold standard.

The major complication of discectomy is failure to relieve pain. Other complications include infection, occurring in about 2 percent of cases; injury to a nerve root or dural laceration, occurring in 1 percent of cases; and recurrent disc herniation.

The third syndrome of lumbar disc disease is cauda equina compression. Occurring acutely, cauda equina compression is a neurosurgical emergency since permanent loss of function can result. Patients with this syndrome typically present with severe back pain, numbness and weakness in the legs, and urinary retention. There is good hope for recovery if timely decompression is done. MRI or myelography show a complete epidural block opposite the disc space. Surgery should include a wide laminectomy of the laminae above and below the lesion and careful removal of the herniated disc.

Occurring chronically, central disc herniation and resultant cauda equina compression produce leg numbness, paresthesias, and low-grade urinary retention. Pain may be deceptively mild and the physical examination may be normal. CT or MRI will establish the disk herniation present in this condition.

The final lumbar disc syndrome is not so much a syndrome of disc disease itself as of its treatment. It is the so-called "failed back" and occurs in a patient who has had one or more disc operations, has often lost his or her job, is taking narcotics, and has tried acupuncture, transcutaneous stimulation, one or more pain clinics, and a variety of other modalities. Typically there is back tenderness, variable pain on straight leg raising, and variable sensory or motor loss on examination. Radiographic studies reveal changes compatible either with scarring and/or arachnoidal adhesions.

Few patients are more difficult to deal with in all of neurosurgery than those with the failed back syndrome. Some guidelines may be helpful: 1) narcotics should not be used; 2) pending lawsuits and compensation cases should be settled before any surgery is considered; 3) although there is a tendency to admit such patients for "one last round" of investigation, it is not clear that this will be productive. A possible assessment of this difficult syndrome can be approached by the following steps: MRI to rule out disc rerupture, nerve blocks to assess roots involved in the pain syndrome, psychiatric consultation to assess the usefulness of antidepressants in pain control, and temporary spinal cord stimulation to assess the usefulness of a permanent epidural spinal cord stumulator. For deafferentation pain clonazepam may be helpful, and tegretol and dilantin are also worth trying. The most consistently helpful medications, however, are the antidepressants. Depression may be a cause of chronic back pain as well as a result. In patients with this syndrome careful history taking seeks out feelings of discouragement, changes in sleep pattern, diminished or increased appetite, fatigue, loss of general interest in life, decreased libido, suicidal feelings, and feelings of worthlessness. If more than five of these are present, the patient is probably experiencing depression and vigorous therapy should be directed toward its alleviation. Despite patients' claims that "you would be depressed if you had this pain," primary treatment of depression can produce remarkable improvement in back pain.

Other Disorders of the Spinal Cord

Several spinal structural abnormalities have neurosurgical implications. *Ankylosing spondylitis,* in which the anterior and posterior longitudinal ligaments calcify, is sometimes associated with severe cord injury after mild trauma because the spine is very brittle and fractures easily. Operative fusion is virtually always required because of consequent instability. *Achondroplastic dwarfism* is commonly associated with spinal stenosis, especially in the lumbar region. *Spondylolysis* is a defect in the pars interarticularis of the lumbar vertebrae. It may be congenital, appearing usually in the teenage years, or may be acquired after trauma. *Spondylolisthesis,* displacement of one vertebral body relative to another, can occur with spondylolysis. L5–S1 is the most common site, causing L5 nerve root entrapment. Surgery requires decompression of the L5 roots and posterolateral fusion; it should be done if radicular pain is significant. In late adult life the same slipping of vertebrae on one another can occur (spondylolisthesis) without spondylolysis. This results from arthritis of the facet joints; decompression and fusion may be indicated if there is more than a 50 percent displacement or a significant neurologic deficit.

Spinal stenosis may affect cervical or lumbar regions; it is a narrowing of the canal so that symptoms of spinal cord or root compression emerge. In the cervical spine, the result is spasticity and sensory loss; in the lumbar spine, a syndrome of "pseudo-claudication" occurs, in which leg pain increases on ambulation.

The diagnosis is made by the clinical history and plain X-rays. In the cervical spine, a distance less than 9 mm at any point in the canal between the posterior plane of a vertebral body and the lamina suggests stenosis. CT appearance of spinal stenosis reveals a trefoil appearance of the spinal canal with hypertrophy of the facet joints.

The treatment is laminectomy of the involved segments plus at least one level above and below. This usually provides very satisfactory relief of the lumbar symptoms. In the neck, recovery from spasticity is less certain but progress of the disease is slowed.

Syringomyelia

Pathologically, syringomyelia is a cavitation and slow accumulation of fluid within the spinal cord. Clinically, it is a syndrome of dissociated sensory loss (i.e., pain lost, light touch preserved) with muscle wasting and weakness beginning in the arms. Causal factors include trauma, arachnoiditis, and Pott's disease. The syndrome can also occur with intraspinal tumors with or without a direct cystic component.

The idiopathic type of syringomyelia occurs in adult life with loss of pain sensation and weakness in the hands because of the arrangement of spinothalamic and corticospinal fibers. There is progressive sensory loss in a "cape" distribution over the shoulders as well as spasticity in the legs. As the syrinx extends higher, there is swallowing trouble and nystagmus. The diagnostic procedure of choice is the MRI. It can demonstrate the widened cord and the cyst within it.

The natural history of a syrinx is slow, steady deterioration. The best surgical approach is still controversial, as is the role of surgery in general. If there is an associated Arnold-Chiari malformation with descent of the tonsils into the foramen magnum, decompression and dural grafting are indicated. If there is no Arnold-

Chiari malformation, the syrinx should be shunted into the subarachnoid space or into the pleural or peritoneal cavity. Other procedures that have been purported to help include ventricular shunting, if there is hydrocephalus, and opening of the dilated central canal to the subarachnoid space in the filum terminale.

Suggestions for Further Reading

Cervical Spine Research Society. *The Cervical Spine*. Second ed. Philadelphia: J.B. Lippincott, 1989.

Kirkaldy-Willis WH and Burton CV. *Managing Low Back Pain*. Third ed. New York: Churchhill Livingston, 1992.

Macnab I and McCulloch J. *Backache*. Second ed. Baltimore: Williams & Wilkins, 1990.

Rothman RH and Simeone FA. *The Spine*. Third ed. Philadelphia: Saunders, 1992.

IV

Special Topics
in Neurosurgery

This last section of the book deals with the management of pediatric neurosurgical patients and the growing subspecialty of stereotactic and functional neurosurgery. Neurosurgical procedures for pain relief and neurological disorders of significance to neurosurgeons will also be discussed.

16

Pediatric Neurosurgery

Neurosurgery in infants and children is different enough from adult neurosurgery to warrant its own neurosurgical subspecialty. This chapter presents a few common syndromes and some specific dis eases that differ substantially in children and adults.

Common Symptoms and Signs in Pediatric Neurosurgery

Macrocephaly

This is a general term meaning "head enlargement." To assess enlargement, the head circumference should be plotted on a percentile chart for height and weight. A circumference consistently above the 97th percentile or 5 mm above it at any age means significant enlargement. Crossing two or more percentile growth lines may indicate abnormal enlargement, except in a premature infant whose head circumference may cross percentile lines in the first 2 months after birth. Conditions causing macrocephaly include hydrocephalus, subdural fluid collection, subdural hematomas, and metabolic diseases including Tay-Sach's and Gaucher's disease. A large head combined with seizures is usually caused by a subdural hematoma.

Seizures

Childhood seizures are similar to adult patterns except that petit mal or absence seizures involving only lapses of attention are more common in children. There are also two patterns peculiar to infants and young children: infantile spasms, which are flexor spasms that resemble tonic seizures, that begin at 3 to 9 months and that generally represent a poor prognosis for normal development; and myoclonic seizures, jerks of an extremity that may be associated with akinesia (falling to the ground).

Children with *major motor seizures* may be suffering from idiopathic epilepsy if they have no focal EEG abnormality and their CT scan is normal. MRI should be ordered to exclude a focal lesion. Phenobarbital is the anticonvulsant drug of choice, used in doses of 3–5 mg/kg per day to keep a serum level of 20–50 ug/ml. Phenytoin alone or in combination with phenobarbital is the drug of second choice, followed by carbamazepine.

"Absence" seizures are characterized by brief losses of consciousness, often with a three-per-second spike and slow waves on the EEG. Most cases (75%) resolve by age 30, especially if they are easily controllable by medication, have no motor component, and begin between ages 4 and 8 years. Ethosuximide (Zarontin) 20–40 mg/kg is the drug of first choice; valproic acid (Depakene) is the second choice but may produce severe liver and blood toxicity.

Myoclonic epilepsy has two major presentations: infantile spasms, with massive flexor spasms of the extremity and trunk associated with hypsarrhythmia of EEG; and late onset myoclonic epilepsy. ACTH 0.40 units/day for 4–6 weeks is the drug of first choice for infantile spasms; a ketogenic diet is often prescribed as well. Valproic acid, clonazepam, or diazepam may also be effective. In late-onset myoclonic epilepsy there are multiple episodes beginning about the age of 1 year, which include jackknife spasms, outward thrusts of the arms with flexion of the trunk (solo arm attacks), akinetic or drop attacks, and absence attacks. The EEG is abnormal. Diseases such as the lipidoses and Lafora's disease should be excluded. Phenobarbital and phenytoin are drugs of first choice.

Five percent of children have febrile seizures, usually between the ages of 6 months and 5 years. Short, sudden seizures with high fever, no focal component, and without a family history of febrile seizures are especially likely to have no long-term sequelae. BUN, electrolytes, sugar Ca, P and Na should be checked, and lumbar puncture may be indicated as well. Immediate management consists of 5 mg/kg phenobarbital IV; prophylactic phenobarbital should be given upon subsequent temperature elevation in patients with previous febrile seizures with any atypical features until they reach the age of 5 years. Long-term prophylaxis may be warranted if the seizures have several atypical features or multiple occurrences.

Ataxia

Acute cerebellar ataxia of childhood may occur after a febrile illness in children between ages 1 and 5 years. Imaging studies are normal and CSF shows a mild lymphocytosis. Other possible causes of acute ataxia in children are intoxication, occult neuroblastoma, maple syrup urine disease, Hartnup's disease, pyruvate decarboxylase deficiency, acute familiar cerebellar ataxia, Guillain Barre syndrome, and benign paroxysmal vertigo. It is important to rule out a posterior fossa tumor or hematoma in all cases of acute ataxia by obtaining a CT or MRI that shows the posterior fossa adequately. Progressive ataxia in children can result from posterior fossa tumor, the ataxia telangiectasia syndrome, abetalipoproteinemia, Refsum's syndrome, and Friedreich's ataxia.

Acute Hemiplegia

Hemiplegia in children less than 3 years of age is usually idiopathic, with seizures as a frequent accompaniment. Intracranial trauma, cardiac emboli, carotid arteritis, sickle cell anemia and other diseases associated with increased blood viscosity, intracranial hemorrhage, and hemiplegic migraine can also cause hemiplegia. In general, a normal CT scan excludes a problem treatable by neurosurgery.

Intellectual Retardation

Progressive intellectual regression in childhood may be caused by any of the diseases listed in Table 16.1. Infantile Gaucher's disease is characterized by a retroflexed head, trismus, and strabismus. Tay-Sach's disease presents with abnormal startle response, seizures, blindness, increased head size, and a cherry-red spot in the macula. Metachromatic leukodystrophy begins as a gait disturbance with later loss of speech and loss of reflexes because of a peripheral neuropathy; seizures are not prominent. Hurler's syndrome is associ-

Table 16.1. Causes of Childhood Intellectual Failure by Age of Onset

Age of Onset	Disorder
Birth	GMI Type 1 gangliosidosis
	Alexander's disease
	Von Gierke's glycogen storage disease
1–3 weeks	Maple syrup urine disease
	Galactosemia
1–3 months	Type 2 storage disease
3–6 months	Gaucher's disease
	Tay-Sach's disease
	Krabbe's disease
	Neimann-Pick disease
	Phenylketonuria
	Amino acid defect
	Canavan's disease
3–12 months	Lesch-Nyhan syndrome
	Pelizaeus-Marzbacher disease
6 months to 2 years	Type 2 GMI gangliocytosis
6 months to 4 years	Homocystinuria
1–3 years	Hurler's syndrome
	Metachromatic leukodystrophy
	Neuroaxonal dystrophy
	Leigh's necrotizing encephalomyelopathy
1–6 years	Neimann-Pick disease
	Late infantile amaurotic idiocy
2–6 years	Hunter's syndrome
	Type 3 gangliosidosis
4–8 years	Juvenile amaurotic idiocy or San Philipo syndrome
5–10 years	Schilder's disease
	Huntington's disease
8–15 years	Myoclonic epilepsy
5–20 years	Juvenile metachromatic leukodystrophy
	Wilson's hepatolenticular degeneration

Adapted from Hoffman and Epstein (1986).

ated with communicating hydrocephalus, dwarf stature, protruberent abdomen, deafness, gargoyle facies, and corneal clouding. Subacute sclerosing panencephalitis (SSPE) begins between the ages of 5 and 15 with slow myoclonic jerks several years after an episode of measles. There is a characteristic burst of supression pattern on EEG.

Specific Disease Entities in Children

This section summarizes several neurological disorders that have different presentation and management in children than in adults.

Head Injuries

Relatively mild head injury in children may be accompanied by sudden massive brain swelling without associated intracranial hematoma. The same problem may occur after head shaking in the child abuse syndrome. Its source appears to be increased cerebral blood volume and its treatment is intubation with hyperventilation. An ICP bolt or other monitoring device is helpful in assessing intracranial pressure. Acute subdural hematomas may occur in children as well as adults; rapid deterioration with coma is a presenting symptom and CT scanning will make the diagnosis, which leads to the emergent evacuation of the hematoma.

Child abuse is one of the major sources of pediatric head trauma. Telltale signs are subdural hematomas of varying age, retinal hemorrhages, and scalp bruises. The body should be examined for bruises elsewhere, and long bone and rib X-rays should be taken to check for fractures incurred at different ages.

In infants up to 2 or 3 years old chronic subdural hematomas are a relatively common problem. These may be associated with convulsions, an enlarged head, vomiting, or retinal hemorrhages. The CT shows low attenuation or isodense collections of fluid around one or both hemispheres. The possibility of child abuse should be kept in mind. Serial subdural taps through the coronal suture are often an effective mode of treatment, although subdural to peritoneal shunting may sometimes be required.

For subdural taps the child is immobilized and the scalp is prepared over the coronal suture. A short, slightly beveled needle (20 gauge) is placed through the coronal suture in line with the pupil or just at the lateral corner. When a pop of the anterior fontanelle is felt, fluid should be allowed to drain under its own pressure until flow ceases. Repeated taps may be required as indicated by the child's condition, the degree of fullness of the anterior fontanelle, and the CT scan.

Spinal Cord Compression in Children

This is a neurosurgical emergency and may present with less clear signs in children than in adults. Back pain, tingling and numbness in the legs, change in urine function, bowel change, or mild weakness are early symptoms and may be confirmed by tenderness over the spine and diminished response to pinprick. This syndrome may be caused by epidural, intradural, or intramedullary masses. Epidural causes in children include epidural abscess or hematoma and metastases of leukemia, lymphoma, or neuroblastoma; intradural causes include neurofibroma, metastatic seeding from a cerebral tumor, or dermoid cyst; and intrinsic spinal cord tumors include astrocytomas and ependymoma. MRI is the initial imaging study of choice. The syndrome of discitis may mimic tumor. It is usually seen in children under age 5 and is associated with severe back pain and spasm, an elevated sedimentation rate, and a normal myelogram.

Myopathies

Weakness in a child with normal reflexes and sensation and with proximal limb strength more impaired than distal suggest a myopathy or dystrophy. Neurological consultation is appropriate.

Brain Tumors

Most brain tumors in children over the age of 2 years occur in the posterior fossa. The most common presentation is that of elevated ICP leading to hydrocephalus and including headache, vomiting, and papilledema; ataxia, diplopia, stiff neck, and head tilt may be associated findings. Cranial nerve palsies and pyramidal tract signs suggest an intrinsic brainstem tumor, most commonly a glioma.

Important childhood tumors include medulloblastoma, ependymoma, cerebellar astrocytoma, and brainstem glioma. Medulloblastomas most commonly occur in the midline in childhood and usually cause hydrocephalus. Extension through the spinal cord pathways is common. These tumors are best treated by excision of as much tumor as is safe followed by radiation therapy, usually to the whole brain and spinal canal.

Cerebellar astrocytomas often present between ages 5 and 10 years and can sometimes be removed completely by surgery. Ependymomas are best treated with surgical extirpation followed by radiation therapy. Brainstem gliomas usually occur from ages 8–15 and present with cranial nerve palsies, cerebellar dysfunction, and hyperreflexia, initially without increased intracranial pressure.

Supratentorial tumors in children include hypothalamic gliomas, which may present with marked body wasting and elevated CSF protein; optic gliomas, which are associated with impaired vision, exophthalmus, optic atrophy, and papilledema; and tumors involving the cerebral hemispheres such as PNET, astrocytic tumors, ependymoma, oligodendroglioma, and ganglioglioma.

Neurocutaneous Syndromes

These include neurofibromatosis, tuberous sclerosis, Sturge-Weber syndrome, and Von Hippel-Landau disease. They are often associated with brain tumors. The most common neurocutaneous syndrome is neurofibromatosis, either type 1, with peripheral nerve lesions primarily or type 2 with CNS lesions. Cutaneous manifestations include cafe-au-lait spots, axillary freckling, Lisch nodules, and subcutaneous neurofibromas. Optic nerve gliomas, bilateral acoustic neuromas, astrocytomas, meningiomas, and spinal cord tumors occur in patients with NF2.

Tuberous sclerosis is characteristically diagnosed by the presence of adenoma sebaceum (a butterfly rash across the nose), mental retardation (in two-thirds of patients), and epilepsy. Shagreen patches (raised plaques in the lumbar region usually seen with a Wood's light), cafe-au-lait spots, and subungual fibromas are associated findings. Retinal nodules may be seen. Parenchymal brain tumors of all kinds are increased along with tumors of the kidneys, heart, and abdominal viscera. The most characteristic brain pathology is subependymal giant cell astrocytoma.

Sturge-Weber syndrome is characterized by a port wine stain of the face and an ipsilateral vascular malformation of the parietal meninges. Contralateral hemiplegia, seizure disorder, and mental retardation are characteristic.

Von Hippel-Lindau disease involves a hemangioblastoma of the cerebellum with a concomitant vascular tumor of the retina. Retinal angiomas may also be associated with brainstem and spinal cord malformations in the Wyburn-Mason syndrome.

Congenital Disorders

This section deals with disorders that begin during in utero development but may not be manifest for many years. They fall into five categories: 1) midline fusion defects in the spine, which include dysraphic states such as myelomeningoceles and encephaloceles, dermal sinuses, spinal lipomas, craniofacial abnormalities, craniovertebral junction anomalies, and certain other disorders of brain formation; 2) craniosynostoses; 3) Arnold-Chiari malformation; 4) hydrocephalus; and 5) chromosomal and metabolic defects.

Disorders of Neural Tube Closure and Early Brain Development

In the spinal column, failure of definitive neural tube closure (spinal dysraphism) leads to a variety of disorders discussed in the next section. In the head and neck, incomplete or poor development leads to anencephaly, in which all or part of the brain fails to form; or an encephalocele, in which a cystic mass containing brain tissue and meninges is found in the neck, occiput, or frontal region. It is important to recognize the latter condition before surgery is done for a nasal or occipital mass. If possible, encephaloceles should be repaired, but this may require major reconstructive effort. Dysplasias of cerebral hemisphere organization include agenesis of the corpus callosum, a condition easily diagnosed by MRI scan that produces few symptoms; holoprosencephaly, in which the chambers of the brain do not form properly; and corpus callosum lipomas, in which fatty tissue is left in the midline of the corpus callosum. Any of these dysplastic cerebral hemisphere disorders may be associated with cleft lip and palate or a widened space between the eyes (hypertelorism). Agyria (lack of gyrus formation) and pachygyria (small abundant abnormal gyri) are deficits of cerebral hemisphere organization and development. Dysplasias of the cerebellar hemisphere include vermian agenesis, a condition with very few symptoms; and the Dandy-Walker malformation, a condition in which a posterior fossa cyst is formed by poor development of CSF outlets and hydrocephalus slowly develops.

This group of developmental abnormalities also includes a series of defects in which parts of the cerebral hemispheres do not form fully: encephalomalacia, where part of a hemisphere shrinks; porencephaly, in which there is a cerebral defect left by a hemorrhage or other mass; and hydranencephaly, in which there is only fluid left in the cranium. These may be the result of an in utero injury rather than defective development.

Craniosynostoses

This group of disorders is characterized by early closure of one or more of the cranial sutures. Sagittal synostosis is most common, producing a long narrow head (scaphocephaly), which can compromise brain development and therefore warrants correction. Rongeuring of bone of the suture and placement of material to prevent reclosure are operative principles in this and other synostoses. Coronal suture closure produces a wide head (brachycephaly), and metopic closure a pointed forehead. Whether these require repair depends on the cosmetic deformity, but surgery is best done in the first year of life if it is going to be done.

Arnold-Chiari Malformation

This anomaly is of importance in both adult and pediatric neurosurgery. It involves downward displacement of the cerebellar tonsils through the foramen magnum. This displacement can be very clearly demonstrated by MRI, which is the imaging modality of choice. Four types were initially described: *Type I,* in which there is lengthening of tonsils through the foramen magnum; this presents in early adult life with diplopia, spastic arm and leg weakness, nystagmus, oscillopsia, lower cranial nerve weakness, and ataxia; *Type II,* a juvenile type always associated with myelomeningocele in which the tonsils, fourth ventricle, medulla, and spinal cord are displaced caudally and kinked; *Type III,* a complete caudal displacement of the cerebellum into the cervical canal; and *Type IV,* a "forme fruste" or occult form of these.

In infants, emergent decompression of the Arnold-Chiari malformation should be performed if the patient presents with respiratory stridor, dysphagia, and other lower brain stem anomalies. In adults, removal of the arch of C1 and the rim of the foramen magnum along with dural grafting may prevent continued deterioration caused by this problem. Hydrocephalus and syringomyelia may be associated with these malformations so shunting is needed in symptomatic cases.

Congenital Hydrocephalus

The term hydrocephalus is usually used to refer to large cerebral ventricles. In infancy it has many causes, the most common being intraventricular hemorrhage. Other infant causes include aqueductal stenosis and abnormal posterior fossa outlet development. It is diagnosed by demonstrating increasing head size, with a head circumference consistently beyond the 97th percentile for several months on growth charts, crossing percentile lines or 5 mm above the 97th percentile at any time. Its suspicion warrants a CT scan or MRI. Physical signs beyond a large head include a bulging anterior fontanel, widened cranial sutures, distended scalp veins, and "setting sun" eyes with markedly increased head size. The differential diagnosis of a large head in infancy includes subdural effusion or subdural hematoma, pseudotumor cerebri, metabolic CNS disease, cerebral gigantism, achondroplasia, and primary megalencephaly.

The CT scan or MRI is diagnostic in hydrocephalus; performing it usually requires general anesthesia in infants. Ultrasound may also show ventricular enlargement in infants with an open fontanel and can be used in place of the CT to avoid radiation exposure.

The treatment of infantile hydrocephalus is ventriculoperitoneal shunting; other techniques are less convenient and less reliable. There are a variety of specific shunt systems, and the most important point about any of them is to use a system that is familiar to the surgeon.

Complications of shunting for infantile hydrocephalus include shunt infection, shunt malfunction, and the slit ventricle syndrome. Shunt infection occurs in 10–20 percent of cases; in ventriculoatrial shunts this may present as bacterial endocarditis or nephritis; after ventriculoperitoneal shunting, shunt malfunctions with low-grade peritoneal infection are often encountered. In these cases the infection is usually staphylococcus epidermidis or other skin organisms known as diphtheroids; virulent infection is uncommon.

Shunt malfunction can be expected to occur at some time in about 60 percent of shunts placed in infancy: headache, vomiting, nausea, and other symptoms of increased intracranial pressure are characteristic of malfunction episodes. Often the syndrome is like a viral illness and only observation or shunt tapping will establish whether it in fact represents malfunction; parents will often know the symptoms well and should be heeded carefully. The CT may reveal enlarged ventricles with malfunction, but ventricular size may not change with a poorly functioning shunt. Shunt tapping should be considered if infection is suspected.

Slit ventricles are peculiar to shunts placed in infancy before fontanel closure. They are characterized by small ventricles that do not change in size despite signs of shunt malfunction. Children may get very ill. The treatment is shunt revision, usually of the ventricular catheter, and placement of a higher pressure valve or antisiphon device.

Chromosome and Metabolic Disorders

Many chromosome and metabolic defects are associated with neurologic syndromes; most of these are of peripheral interest to the neurosurgeon. Lipid storage diseases such as Tay-Sachs and Gaucher's, however, and metachromatic leukodystrophy may present with a large head (macrocephaly) mimicking hydrocephalus.

Congenital Disorders of the Spinal Column

Spinal Congenital Disorders

A variety of developmental abnormalities may affect the bony spinal canal; many of them have importance to the neurosurgeon. Three such disorders are spina bifida occulta, block vertebrae (known as hemivertebrae), and the Klippel-Feil abnormality. Spina bifida occulta is characterized by laminae failing to form over one portion of the spinal canal, and it is an important anomaly to recognize before exposing the spinal canal surgically. In block vertebrae there is fusion of two or more adjacent vertebral bodies; this is important because increased stress is placed on the adjacent bodies and may place the patient at increased risk for injury during sports or other vigorous activities. In the Klippel-Fiel abnormality, block vertebrae in the cervical region are associated with a short thick neck.

Among the other developmental disorders that directly involve the spinal cord are the dysraphic states, a series of disorders of neural tube closure that range from rachiscisis (complete exposure of the canal) to dermal tracts in the lumbar region.

Myelomeningoceles

A myelomeningocele is one type of defect in the formation of the neural tube, the embryological precursor of both the spinal column and spinal cord. In its most severe form there may be a complete lack of spinal cord formation. A meningocele involves only bony and meningeal abnormalities; a myelomeningocele involves spinal cord, meninges, and bone; and an encephalocele involves the brain and its coverings. The cause of these defects is unclear.

Prenatal diagnosis is facilitated by elevated alpha-feta protein levels in amniotic fluid and variably in maternal serum. This is an accurate method of screening, and ultrasound can usually provide the definitive diagnosis. At birth, the myelomeningocele is readily established by physical examination, disclosing an epithelial defect in the midline with a clear cystic excrescence containing neural tissue in the midline. An important issue is what movement is possible below the abnormality.

Currently in the United States aggressive treatment is indicated for infants with these congenital abnormalities. Such treatment involves closure of the defect within the first 72 hours to avoid meningitis, shunting for hydrocephalus either at the same time or as soon as it can conveniently be done, orthopedic and urologic procedures as necessary to maintain maximum function, and treatment of all infections with appropriate antibiotics. The longterm outlook for children with this disorder depends on the severity of their neurologic deficit as well as their home support and their medical care.

Suggestions for Further Reading

Hoffman HJ and Epstein F. *Disorders of the Developing Nervous System: Diagnosis and Treatment*. Boston: Blackwell Scientific, 1986.
Raimondi AJ. *Pediatric Neurosurgery*. New York: Springer-Verlag, 1987.
Rekate HL. *Comprehensive Management of Spina Bifida*. Boca Raton, Fla.: CRC Press, 1991.
Shillito J Jr and Matson DD. *An Atlas of Pediatric Neurosurgical Operations*. Philadelphia: W.B. Saunders, 1982.

17

Stereotactic and Functional Neurosurgery

Stereotactic neurosurgery is done by using three-dimensional guidance coordinates. With its recent coupling to CT scan and to MRI, stereotactic surgery is witnessing a resurgence that is one of the most important developments in contemporary neurosurgery. Stereotactic procedures are done for three general reasons: to biopsy and perhaps remove deep-seated tumors or tumors of difficult access, to help manage selected movement disorders, and to manage some chronic pain states.

Several devices are now widely available. The three most commonly used are the Cosman-Roberts-Wells, Brown-Roberts-Wells, and Leksell frames. They all establish coordinates with either intracranial or extracranial landmarks and then use a guidance system for delivering a probe to the target based on its relationship to these coordinates. Most stereotactic neurosurgery can be done with the patient awake.

Tumor Biopsy and Treatment

Intracranial lesions amenable to stereotactic biopsy include those deeply seated in the thalamus or basal ganglia; those beneath such important regions of the cortex as primary sensory and motor areas, visual receptive areas, and speech areas; and those that may be hard to localize at open operation even if they are in "silent" areas. Posterior fossa lesions, pontine, and medullary lesions are risky to approach stereotactically unless they are cystic; biopsy of very vascular lesions should not be attempted. In centers where these techniques are used routinely, however, especially with the CRW frame, highly vascular lesions may be safely biopsied, suggesting that any mass lesion in the brain should be considered for biopsy before radiation or other potentially neurotoxic treatments are used. The major risk is hemorrhage, which occurs in 1 percent of cases.

Stereotactic techniques can also be used for definitive treatment of brain tumors by surgical or laser extirpation. Temporary implantation of high-activity radiation sources can deliver large dosages to the tumor and much less to the surrounding brain. The isotope cannulas are inserted to fit the three-dimensional volume of tumor described by the CT scan. Stereotactic techniques can be coupled with conventional surgery to remove lesions as well. Full craniotomy can be done in the stereotactic frame to protect eloquent areas such as cortex controlling speech or movement. For small lesions, laser vaporization can be used with microscopic and stereotactic control.

A new and exciting application of stereotaxis is stereotactic radiosurgery, in which X-ray beams are focused on an intracranial target. This is extremely important in the management of inaccessible vascular malformations, metastatic tumors, and some other tumors. These should be less than 5 cm in size.

Functional Neurosurgery

Functional neurosurgery is done to modify brain function rather than to remove abnormal tissue; it is primarily used to treat tremor or other movement disorders, epilepsy, and pain.

Tremor and Other Movement Disorders

Tremor is the movement disorder most responsive to stereotactic ablation techniques, although some centers report good results with dystonia as well. Ventrolateral thalamotomy is the procedure used in most cases. The region of the thalamus to be destroyed is located anatomically by relating it to the anterior and posterior commissures of the thalamus and physiologically by measuring the effects of skin touch on thalamic electrical activity. In general, standard radiological techniques, including ventriculography, are still used for these procedures; however, MRI may become the procedure of choice in the future.

The tremor of Parkinson's disease is abolished in 85–90 percent of cases; rigidity is helped in 80 percent. Bradykinesia is not helped. As pharmacological management of Parkinson's disease is often ineffective after 5 years, there may be an increasing place for thalamotomy in the future. Other movement disorders may also be helped; essential tremor that is refractory to inderal responds in 80 percent of cases, and dystonia musculorum deformans and atheotosis of cerebral palsy both have varying responses.

Pallidotomy is also used presently in Parkinson's disease.

Epilepsy

Seizure surgery is being more widely practiced as it becomes clear that it is safe and effective. It is still reserved for cases that fail medical therapy, however. There are two fundamental kinds of operation to treat epilepsy—resection of epileptogenic tissue and callosotomy: There are also two procedures for identifying and measuring electrical activity—subdural electrodes and implanted "depth" electrodes.

To evaluate a seizure focus, long-term monitoring with scalp electrodes is the first step. PET scanning may also be helpful, and MRI should be done at least once if there is a focal component to seizures. Any patient with seizures occurring for the first time in adult life should have an MRI or CT scan.

If scalp electrodes do not demonstrate a focus satisfactorily, consideration may be given to invasive monitoring with subdural or depth electrodes. Subdural electrodes require a craniotomy and are best if superficial sites are suspected; depth electrodes are more precise but penetrate the brain.

If a focus is demonstrated electrically, consideration may be given to its resection if medical therapy with anticonvulsants fails to control seizures adequately. Resection may be of focal tissue (topectomy), of an epileptogenic lobe (temporal—frontal lobectomy), or of the whole hemisphere (hemispherectomy). For this and other surgical decisions in epilepsy, a team is required.

Temporal lobectomy has a very high rate of improving seizures, with 80 percent of patients showing some improvement, 60 percent seizure-free on medication, and 20 percent able to come off medication. Frontal lobectomy and topectomy have less effect. Hemispherectomy has a very high success rate.

Division of the corpus callosum is used almost exclusively for drop attacks in which patients will suddenly fall and injure themselves. Callosotomy can be partial or complete; if it is complete a syndrome of chronic disconnection is possible, but in patients selected for this procedure this is not apparent because of their developmental delay. Callosotomy has a 60 percent chance of improving seizures.

Neurosurgery for Pain Relief

The Pathophysiology of Pain

The neurosurgical understanding of pain pathways has evolved from a belief that simple tracts transmit "pain" impulses from periphery to brain, to a much more complex understanding of efferent and afferent sensory systems subserving the perception of pain. Our current understanding may be very briefly summarized as follows. Stimuli are transmitted from simple cutaneous nerve endings by A and C fibers in peripheral nerves to the dorsal horn of the spinal cord. Neurons of the dorsal horn send axons to the spinothalamic tract, which crosses midline within one or two vertebral levels above the nerve root that carried the stimulus. This tract travels to the ventrolateral nucleus of the thalamus and then projects to sensory cortex; however, about 75 percent of spinothalamic fibers synapse with interneurons to form a slow pathway to the nuclei medullooblongata centralis, and another pathway through periaqueductal and periventricular gray to the centromedian and parafascicular nuclei, and thence to the intralaminar nucleus of the thalamus. An important discovery has been that efferent pathways from the brainstem travel to the spinal cord with the likely function of suppressing apparently painful stimuli. It therefore becomes possible to imagine enhancement of these pathways as a means of intrinsic control of pain.

Manipulation at the Level of the Spinal Cord to Control Pain

Spinal cord manipulation is used primarily to relieve pain in the limbs. *Dorsal column stimulation* aroused great interest when it was first introduced. Currently, there has been limited interest in this procedure, which involves placement of electrodes in the epidural space over the spinal cord. It appears to be most useful in paients with unilateral lower extremity pain secondary to chronic radiculopathy.

Two procedures attempt to relieve pain by ablation of spinal cord neurons or tracts. *Dorsal root entry zone* (DREZ) lesions are made in the spinal cord and destroy Rexed areas I-V. The procedure is most efficacious when used to treat pain secondary to nerve root avulsion or spinal cord injury. *Cordotomy* is the destruction of a spinothalamic tract to prevent transmission of pain impulses. It is useful for unilateral pain from cancer, but its effect tends to wear off within 2 years. It is not effective in causalgia, rectal or bladder cancer pain, dysesthetic (deep burning) pain, or Charcot joint pain.

There are two cordotomy techniques, open and percutaneous. In the open technique, a laminectomy is done, the dentate ligaments are identified, and an incision is made in the spinal cord anterior to the dentate ligament. If the pain is below the midthorax, the cordotomy is done at the level of T1–2; if it involves the anus, it is done at lower lumbar levels.

Epidural morphine administration is an important new technique for the relief of pain of spinal origin (cancer pain, arachnoiditis). An epidural catheter is implanted under fluoroscopic control and tested by intermittent injection of 1 mg morphine every 24 hours. If this produces pain relief over a 7–8 day period, the catheter is implanted subcutaneously and connected either to a subcutaneous refillable catheter or to a subcutaneous infusion pump. Respiratory depression is an important potential complication.

Treating Pain at the Level of the Peripheral Nerve or Dorsal Root

Two procedures are often used in attempts to relieve pain at the level of the peripheral nerve or root: transcutaneous stimulation and posterior rhizotomy. Transcutaneous stimulation is often the first line of treatment for this type of pain syndrome. It can give good relief for 1 to 3 days, but has a long-term success rate of only about 35 percent. In this technique, a patient applies flat metal electrodes along the skin surface over the nerves affected and uses a variety of amplitudes and frequencies of electrical pulses. Its principle is to "close the pain gate." It is most useful for stump and phantom limb pain, postherpetic neuralgia, and nerve injury. It has generally not been helpful in pain from peripheral neuropathy, from spinal cord injury, or of thalamic origin.

Dorsal rhizotomy can be done either by open surgery or by percutaneous radiofrequency ablation. If laminectomy is used, it is usually necessary to cut the roots above and below the root apparently affected. In radiofrequency rhizotomy the electrode is placed percutaneously, usually with wake-up anesthesia or under local anesthesia to assure appropriate sensory and motor response to test stimulation. In either case, preoperative nerve block testing does not appear to predict accurately the effect of rhizotomy.

Treating Pain at the Level of the Brain

A recent use for stereotactic surgery is the implantation of electrodes to stimulate the brain in chronic pain states. The sensory relay nucleus of the thalamus (nucleus ventralis posterior) and periaqueductal and periventricular gray matter are the target areas. This technique is still in its infancy. Similarly, cingulotomy, which uses ventricular outlines for its coordinates, is a promising but still uncertain technique in neurosurgery for pain. It appears to be remarkably effective when pain complicates an intractable depression, without measurable cognitive defects.

Stereotactic techniques have been applied to pituitary ablation for chronic pain due to endocrine-sensitive malignancy. Done under general anesthesia they involve radiofrequency heating or cooling of the gland and are an effective means of destroying the pituitary. They will give pain relief in roughly 80 percent of breast cancer patients and 70 percent of prostate cancer patients, and will produce a remission of the tumor in a smaller percentage of cases.

Management of Trigeminal Neuralgia

As noted above, there has been a move away from the simple concept that interrupting a pain transmission pathway will relieve pain; however, there are several neurosurgical ablative procedures that do have varying degrees of success.

Trigeminal neuralgia (tic douloreaux) is characterized by paroxysmal episodes of lancinating facial pain in one or more divisions of the trigeminal nerve; there is usually a trigger point that will reproduce the pain. Examination usually reveals no sensory loss and may reproduce pain on touching a trigger point. There is some evidence that the pathologic mechanism is compression of the poorly myelinated root entry zone of the trigeminal nerve by an artery or vein. Carbamazepine up to 800 mg a day, or to the point of neurologic toxicity (drowsiness, staggering, vertigo), is the initial treatment of choice; if this does not work, some physicians have suggested a trial of phenytoin for 2 to 3 months. It is important to follow the white blood cell count regularly while a patient is on carbamazepine since bone marrow suppression can be a lethal side effect.

At present there are two surgical approaches to trigeminal neuralgia. The first is a retrogasserian injury to the sensory fibers subserving trigeminal pain by radiofrequency lesioning, glycerol injections, or balloon compression. In radiofrequency heating, the patient reports on the degree of sensory loss to allow destruction of pain fibers without destruction of sensory fibers that affect the corneal reflex. An electrode is inserted through a spinal needle under radiographic guidance to enter the foramen ovale at the base of the brain and extend beyond it to the root entry zone of the trigeminal nerve. With this technique there is good pain relief in 80–90 percent of cases. The major complication is called "anesthesia dolorosa," a painful condition that is difficult to treat. The second technique is to inject 5 cc of 99.9 percent glycerol to ablate some of the pain-subserving fibers; this is placed by the same techniques as retrogasserian rhizotomy with care to avoid passage out of the ganglion.

The other surgical approach used with considerable success in trigeminal neuralgia is decompression of the trigeminal root entry zone in the posterior fossa. The rationale for this procedure is that compression of the nerve by an artery loop may be the primary cause of trigeminal neuralgia. In approximately 85 percent of cases, patients have an obvious compressive lesion, and a decompressive procedure that involves suboccipital craniectomy and moving the artery off the nerve gives complete relief. There is a mortality rate of 0.5 percent with this procedure.

Suggestions for Further Reading

Bonica JJ. *The Management of Pain*. Second ed. Philadelphia: Lea & Febiger, 1990.

Kelly PJ. *Tumor Stereotaxis*. Philadelphia: W.B. Saunders, 1991.

Spencer SS and Spencer DD. *Surgery for Epilepsy*. Cambridge, Mass.: Blackwell, 1991.

18

Selected Neurological Disorders of Neurosurgical Importance

By the nature of the subject, the student of neurosurgery is also a student of neurology, and must recognize all types of neurological illnesses. This chapter presents five neurological disorders that can mimic neurosurgical disorders and should be recognized in this guise.

Alzheimer's Disease and Other Dementias

Alzheimer's disease is a common degenerative disease of the brain that must be distinguished from normal pressure hydrocephalus. Progressive generalized failure of cognitive processes is characteristic of Alzheimer's disease; motor signs are uncommon as an early manifestation. Normal pressure hydrocephalus, on the other hand, presents with walking difficulty as a major, early sign in most cases that would improve with shunting. Several other treatable conditions can cause dementia and should be excluded by the appropriate testing in an elderly patient with dementia: thyroid testing to exclude myxedema, B12 levels to exclude pernicious anemia, CSF serology to exclude syphilis, CT scan with contrast to exclude a brain tumor, a family history to check for Huntington's disease, and an electroencephalogram to differentiate Alzheimer's from Jakob-Creutzfeld disease. Perhaps the hardest differential diagnosis to rule out is depression, which may require prolonged observation and perhaps a trial of antidepressants. Pick's disease is much rarer than Alzheimer's disease, with primarily frontal and temporal atrophy and a clinical and pathological picture resembling Alzheimer's.

Parkinson's Disease

Parkinson's disease is important in neurosurgery because of the possibility of using thalamotomy or pallidotomy to treat its characteristic tremor. In Parkinson's disease dopamine is depleted in the caudate nucleus, putamen, and globus pallidum because nigrostriatal dopaminergic neurons degenerate. As a result, cholinergic input to the basal ganglia is unchecked. The classical clinical triad consists of tremor, rigidity, and bradykinesia. Disturbances of posture, equilibrium, and autonomic function as well as depression are also common. The tremor can be extremely variable but is usually of the "pill-rolling" type. The body posture is characteristic with head bowed, trunk bent, shoulders dropped, and the arms flexed at the elbow.

The cause of Parkinson's disease is unknown. Its symptoms can be associated with carbon monoxide poisoning, heavy metal intoxication, brain tumors of the basal ganglia, some infections, cerebral arteriosclerosis, hypoparathyroidism, and phenothiazine use. There are several variants of Parkinsonism, and in Guam there is a complex of Parkinsonism, dementia, and amyotrophic lateral sclerosis that appears to be genetically based. Progressive supranuclear palsy consists of Parkinsonism, mental disturbance, and profound impairment first of downward and later of upward gaze.

Drug therapy of Parkinsonism includes levodopa, which increases dopamine synthesis; it is contraindicated in patients with hemolytic anemia, glucose-6-phosphate dehydrogenase deficiency, or melanoma. It is usually given with a dopa decarboxylase inhibitor that enhances its effect. Five to six grams of levodopa daily is the average optimal dose. Other agents include anticholinergics, which block reuptake of monoamines at the synaptic cleft.

Parkinsonian tremor should be differentiated from essential tremor. The latter is rhythmical, regular, and more rapid; it is often suppressed by alcohol. Inderal may help in its management. In the elderly a fine rapid tremor of voluntary movement is common.

Friedreich's Ataxia

Friedreich's ataxia is important to the neurosurgeon as a cause of ataxia and extensor plantar response. It is a genetic disorder whose mode of transmission is unclear. Ataxia (especially in young adults), muscle weakness, posterior column findings, absent reflexes, club feet, and scoliosis are characteristic. Cardiac murmur and cardio-megaly are common associated findings. Other forms of cerebellar degeneration include hereditary cerebellar ataxia, olivopontocere-bellar atrophy, and parenchymatous cerebellar degeneration.

Amyotrophic Lateral Sclerosis

Amyotrophic lateral sclerosis (ALS) is a disease of motor neurons of the brain and spinal cord involving atrophy and weakness of muscles and degeneration of descending spinal tracts. Its clinical presentation is typically weakness and atrophy of muscles with fibrillation and fasciculations and with an increase in deep tendon reflexes. Muscle pains occur in 50 percent of cases, and urinary symptoms in 15–20 percent. Life expectancy is 5 years after onset.

Polyneuritis, multiple sclerosis, spinal cord tumor, syringomyelia, osteoarthritis of the cervical spine, cervical ribs, and muscular atrophy may all present clinically similar pictures. Sensory changes usually accompany spinal cord compression and syringomyelia; myelography or MRI will exclude these.

Multiple Sclerosis

Multiple sclerosis is characterized by a variety of neurologic symptoms and signs tending to remit and exacerbate. Its symptoms are so diverse as to reflect injury to any part of the neuroaxis; multifocality and varying degrees of severity are characteristic. The most common areas affected are the optic chiasm, brainstem, and posterior columns. More than three-quarters of patients with this disease have occular disturbance, muscle weakness, spasticity, and hyperreflexia, Babinski sign, absent abdominal reflexes, dysmetria, and retention or urinary disturbance at some time. Diagnosis requires lesions separated by both location and time.

Clinical guidelines for the diagnosis of multiple sclerosis reflect the dissemination of lesions over time and space. The globulin of CSF is increased with a selective increase in oligoclonal bands of IGG. Syphilis, postinfectious myelopathies, and subacute sclerosing panencephalitis may show similar IGG elevations. Visual and auditory evoked responses are helpful, showing abnormalities in 70 percent of patients. The MRI is the most helpful radiographic test, showing multiple areas of low signal. The ultimate diagnosis must rest on the occurrence of lesions involving different parts of the nervous system over long periods of time.

Suggestions for Further Reading

Adams RD and Victor M. *Principles of Neurology*. Fourth ed. New York: McGraw-Hill, 1989.
Rowland LP. *Merritt's Textbook of Neurology*. Eighth ed. Philadelphia: Lea & Febiger, 1989.
Samuels MA. *Manual of Neurology: Diagnosis and Therapy*. Fourth ed. Boston: Little, Brown, 1991.

INDEX